A NURSE'S
SURVIVAL GUIDE TO
MENTORING

Titles in this series:
Richards & Edwards: A Nurse's Survival Guide to the Ward
Richards: A Nurse's Survival Guide to Drugs in Practice
Thomas: A Nurse's Survival Guide to Leadership and Management on the Ward
Edwards & Sabato: A Nurse's Survival Guide to Critical Care
Elcock & Sharples: A Nurse's Survival Guide to Mentoring
Harrison & Daly: A Nurse's Survival Guide to Acute Medical Emergencies
Fraser & Cooper: A Survival Guide to Midwifery

Commissioning Editor: Mairi McCubbin
Development Editor: Sheila Black
Project Manager: Nayagi Athmanathan
Designer: Charles Gray
Illustration Manager: Merlyn Harvey
Illustrator: David Banks

2 JUN 2012

A NURSE'S

SURVIVAL GUIDE TO

MENTORING

Karen Elcock BSc MSc PGDip CertEd(FE) RN RNT FHEA

Director of Practice and Work-based Learning, Practice Education Support
Unit, Thames Valley University, London, UK

Kath Sharples BN MA PGDip PGCert RN RNT

Senior Lecturer – Learning Community Education Advisor, Practice Education
Support Unit, Thames Valley University, London, UK

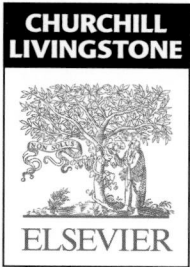

CHURCHILL
LIVINGSTONE

ELSEVIER

EDINBURGH   LONDON   NEW YORK   OXFORD   PHILADELPHIA
ST LOUIS   SYDNEY   TORONTO   2011

CHURCHILL
LIVINGSTONE
ELSEVIER

ISBN 978-0-7020-3946-1
Reprinted 2011

British Library Cataloguing in Publication Data
A catalogue record for this book is available from the British Library

Library of Congress Cataloging in Publication Data
A catalog record for this book is available from the Library of Congress

Notices
Knowledge and best practice in this field are constantly changing. As new research and experience broaden our understanding, changes in research methods, professional practices, or medical treatment may become necessary.

Practitioners and researchers must always rely on their own experience and knowledge in evaluating and using any information, methods, compounds, or experiments described herein. In using such information or methods they should be mindful of their own safety and the safety of others, including parties for whom they have a professional responsibility.

With respect to any drug or pharmaceutical products identified, readers are advised to check the most current information provided (i) on procedures featured or (ii) by the manufacturer of each product to be administered, to verify the recommended dose or formula, the method and duration of administration, and contraindications. It is the responsibility of practitioners, relying on their own experience and knowledge of their patients, to make diagnoses, to determine dosages and the best treatment for each individual patient, and to take all appropriate safety precautions.

To the fullest extent of the law, neither the Publisher nor the authors, contributors, or editors, assume any liability for any injury and/or damage to persons or property as a matter of products liability, negligence or otherwise, or from any use or operation of any methods, products, instructions, or ideas contained in the material herein.

ELSEVIER your source for books, journals and multimedia in the health sciences

www.elsevierhealth.com

Working together to grow
libraries in developing countries

www.elsevier.com | www.bookaid.org | www.sabre.org

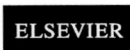
ELSEVIER   BOOK AID International   Sabre Foundation

The Publisher's policy is to use **paper manufactured from sustainable forests**

Printed in China

Contents

Contributors   xi
Preface   xiii

Chapter 1
Mentoring Today   1
Mentoring and nursing   1
Your experience as a student   1
Knowing how it feels   3
Mentorship and professional development   4
Mentoring and recruitment   5
Mentoring for success   6

Chapter 2
Mentoring and the NMC   7
The NMC standards for learning and assessment in practice   7
What are the standards?   8
Becoming a mentor   10
The local mentor register   12
Mentor updating   14
The triennial review and mentor portfolio   18
Applying due regard   20
The sign-off mentor – a brief introduction   22
The mentor's role and responsibility   23

Chapter 3
Preparing for Students   29
Before the student arrives   29
Student expectations   29
Is your practice area prepared?   30
What can go wrong?   31
Creating a learning environment   33

Personal preparation   35
General planning   38
Preparation of resources   44
Getting student preparation right   47
Preparation is the key   48

Chapter 4
Understanding the Practice Assessment
Document   51
The practice assessment document   51
Documenting assessment   53
Learning contracts   54
Using the practice assessment document during placement   55
Writing in the pad   56
Learning outcomes   57
Translating the jargon   60
Identification of learning opportunities   60
Evidence   62
Pulling it altogether   63
Assessing in practice   67

Chapter 5
Orientation and the Initial Interview   69
Meeting your student   69
Orientation   69
Initial interview   71
Learning styles   75
Practice learning outcomes   79
Ongoing achievement record   79
Planning learning experiences   80
Disclosure of a disability   81
Expectations of competence   82
Scheduling feedback   85
Personality clashes   85
Understanding the documentation   86
Making the most of the initial interview   87

Chapter 6
Giving Feedback   89
Feedback   89
Previous experience of feedback   90
Assessment and feedback   91
Informal feedback   94
Formal feedback   95
Delivering feedback   96
Constructive feedback   98
Feedback and self-esteem   99
The feedback sandwich   99
Documenting feedback   101
Difficult feedback   103
Documenting the ongoing achievement record   105
Fair and honest feedback   105

Chapter 7
The Midpoint Interview   107
What is the purpose of the midpoint interview?   107
When should the interview take place?   108
Responsibility for the midpoint interview   114
Feedback at the midpoint interview   115
Measuring progress at the midpoint   119
Documenting at the midpoint interview   120
Action planning   122
Seeking help at the midpoint interview   124
Making the most of the midpoint interview   125

Chapter 8
Supporting the Failing Student   127
What do we mean by failing?   127
Mentoring challenges – the failing student   127
Do not avoid failing students   128
What is the student failing?   128
Why is my student failing?   130
Discussing competence with students   133
Giving feedback to failing students   136

Early failure does not mean end failure 137
Helping failing students 138
Getting help for failing students 140
Don't forget to document 141
Making the final assessment decision 142
What happens when a student does not pass? 145
Did I fail? 147

Chapter 9
The Final Interview 149
The end of placement 149
What is the point of a final interview? 149
Final interview checklist 150
Content of the final interview 151
Completing the final interview and assessment 155
Documentation in the final interview 158
Failing the final assessment 160
The failing mentor 165
Ending on a high note 165
Reflection on your experience 166
Improving your own standard of mentoring 166

Chapter 10
The Role of the Sign-off Mentor 167
What is a sign-off mentor? 167
How do I become a sign-off mentor? 168
Preparing for your role as sign-off mentor 176
Supporting others 176
Making time to meet with your student 177
The ongoing achievement record 178
Self-assessment – am I ready? 182

Chapter 11
Mentoring Students with Disabilities 185
Introduction 185
Models of disability 186
Disability and the law 188
Disability and the NMC 191

The implications of the DDA for the mentor   192
Disclosure   193
Reasonable adjustments for specific impairments or disabilities   200
Assessing the disabled student   205
Evaluating your support of the student with a disability   206

Chapter 12
Mentoring Challenges   209
Introduction   209
Mentoring students on a second attempt   209
The work–life balance   214
Professional conduct   217
Sickness and absenteeism   220
Incidents/accidents   221
Pregnancy   221
Motivating students   223
Student complaints   224
Managing a crossover of student placements   226
Refusing care from students   227
Involving other services/teams   228
Mentoring in different types of placement areas   229
Where to find help   232

Chapter 13
Using Simulated Learning   233
What is simulated learning?   233
Why use simulation   234
Using simulation in nurse education   234
Simulation in clinical practice   235
Provision of simulated learning   235
Types of simulation   236
Are you and your area prepared for simulated learning?   238
Planning effective simulation   239
Information for simulated patient   243
Feedback forms   244
Personal preparation   247
Debriefing as part of simulation   249
Planning for feedback   250
Delivering feedback   252

Students' attitudes to simulation 253
Getting it right 254

Chapter 14
Evaluating the Learning Experience 257
Why evaluation is important 257
When to evaluate 257
What to evaluate 258
The student's experience of the placement 258
The quality of the placement as a learning environment 259
Evaluating your own experience 263
Analysing evaluations 266
Lessons learnt 269
Improving the learning environment 270
Positive mentoring 272

Appendix
The developmental framework to support learning and assessment in practice 273

Index 285

Contributors

Audrey Blenkharn BSc(Hons) MSc DipLSN RCNT RGN
Senior Lecturer/Programme Leader, Faculty of Health and Human Sciences,
Thames Valley University, London, UK

Chapter 7 *The midpoint interview*

Deann Cox BSc
Senior Lecturer, Simulation Centre,
Thames Valley University, London,UK

Chapter 13 *Using simulated learning*

Karen Elcock BSc MSc PGDip CertEd(FE) RN RNT FHEA
Director of Practice and Work-based Learning, Practice Education Support Unit,
Thames Valley University, London, UK

Chapter 2 *Mentoring and the NMC*

Chapter 10 *The role of the sign-off mentor*

Chapter 11 *Mentoring students with disabilities*

Chapter 14 *Evaluating the learning experience*

Sharon Elliott BA(Hons) MSc RCNT RN
Senior Lecturer, Simulation Centre,
Thames Valley University, London, UK

Chapter 13 *Using simulated learning*

Melanie Gasston-Hales BSc(Hons) Thorn MA RN-MH RNT
Senior Lecturer/Learning Community Education Advisor, Practice Education
Support Unit, Thames Valley University, London, UK

Chapter 4 *Understanding the practice assessment document*

Chapter 12 *Mentoring challenges*

Karen Murrell BA(Hons) MSc RGN
Head of Simulation, School of Nursing, Midwifery and Healthcare, Faculty of
Health and Human Sciences, Thames Valley University, London

Chapter 13 *Using simulated learning*

Kath Sharples BN MA PGDip PGCert RN RNT
Senior Lecturer – Learning Community Education Advisor, Practice
Education Support Unit, Thames Valley University, UK

Chapter 1 Mentoring today

Chapter 3 Preparing for students

Chapter 5 Orientation and the initial interview

Chapter 6 Giving feedback

Chapter 8 Supporting the failing student

Chapter 9 The final interview

PREFACE

There are currently thousands of nurses in the UK with mentor qualifications supporting, guiding and facilitating the learning experiences of pre-registration nursing students. Mentors are the unsung heroes of our profession; tirelessly supporting the development of novice practitioners and contributing their wealth of knowledge, skill and professionalism to ensure nursing remains a respected and highly valued profession. Our intention in writing this book was to provide a valuable resource for those who are already qualified mentors, as it will clarify the various issues and roles that are an integral part of your accountability and responsibility. If you are unsure of your role, or perhaps have become 'stale' as a mentor, then this book will help to motivate and inspire you to reach your full potential. If you would like to build and improve on skills that you already have then this book will help you to identify specific strategies that you can incorporate into your current practice. If you have identified areas that are not working for you in your mentoring role then this book will help you to clarify and rectify your current practice.

WHAT IF I'M NOT A MENTOR?

This book will also be useful for those who are contemplating developing their careers by undertaking a mentorship course. The realities and challenges of the role will be clearly presented, with insights into the opportunities and challenges that you will face as a mentor. If you are considering becoming a mentor then we ask first and foremost that you do so because you want to make a positive impact on the learning experience of students on practice placement. This book will help you to uncover exactly what that impact can be and also elaborate and explain where the mentoring role fits in terms of professional accountability and responsibility.

USING THE BOOK

First and foremost, this book is designed to be a user-friendly, accessible resource for qualified mentors and those interested in finding out more about the role. It can either be read cover to cover, or read in a sequence that meets an individual interest and need. All chapters provide both case studies and activities that offer an opportunity to review realistic mentoring issues within a practice placement context. In addition, we have provided key points and top tips throughout the book to highlight specific advice related to the mentoring role. At all stages of the book you are encouraged to reflect on your own practice in relation to the current standards of mentorship in the UK.

STANDARDS OF MENTORSHIP

The Nursing and Midwifery Council (NMC) *Standards to Support Learning and Assessment in Practice* (2008) provide a standard that all mentors must meet in order to support and assess students on programmes which lead to registration or a recordable qualification on the NMC register. This book has been written in support of these standards. As a result, this book may also be used by qualified mentors to reflect and update themselves on the current standards required of them by the NMC. While each chapter addresses a particular theme related to mentoring, it also supports a number of specific criteria within the NMC standards.

MAPPING THE NMC STANDARDS TO THIS BOOK

We have therefore decided to summarize this book both in terms of content of each chapter and also the specific NMC standards that each chapter will support if relevant. In many cases one NMC standard will be applicable to a number of chapters. As a quick resource this mapping exercise may help to clarify specific chapters that may be of immediate interest to you. However, we have also provided the full version of the NMC standards at the end of the book (see Appendix) so you can view them in their totality.

CHAPTER 1

The purpose of Chapter 1 is to develop an understanding of the student's experience of mentorship. The chapter provides an opportunity to reflect on your own experiences of mentorship and discuss the difference that mentorship can make for students to the placement experience. You will also be able to identify the benefits of mentorship in terms of professional development and recruitment

CHAPTER 2

The aim of Chapter 2 is to provide an insight into the current *Standards to Support Learning and Assessment in Practice* (2008) set by the NMC for mentorship. If you are not familiar with these standards then this chapter will provide a quick introduction to the key points relating to mentorship in the NMC's Standards. You will also be able to undertake a self-assessment of your knowledge, skills and competence against the NMC's developmental framework for mentors and develop an action plan to address any deficiencies. In so doing you will also develop a portfolio of evidence to demonstrate you meet the NMC's standards for mentors.

Box P.1 Mapping Chapter 2 to the NMC standards

- Demonstrate an understanding of factors that influence how students integrate into practice settings
- Be accountable for confirming that students have met or not met the NMC competencies in practice and as a sign-off mentor confirm that students have met or not met the NMC standards of proficiency and are capable of safe and effective practice
- Participate in self and peer evaluation to facilitate personal development and contribute to the development of others
- Contribute to strategies to increase or review the evidence base used to support practices
  (NMC, 2008)

CHAPTER 3

The aim of Chapter 3 is to explore the preparation that may be required prior to mentoring a student. The chapter highlights the key elements of a learning environment, and provides an opportunity to evaluate your own strengths and weaknesses in terms of your personal preparation for students. The chapter is designed to allow an opportunity to plan effectively for a student's arrival.

Box P.2 Mapping Chapter 3 to the NMC standards

- Demonstrate an understanding of factors that influence how students integrate into practice settings
- Identify aspects of the learning environment which could be enhanced negotiating with others to make appropriate changes
- Contribute to the development of an environment in which effective practice is fostered, implemented, evaluated and disseminated
- Initiate and respond to practice developments to ensure safe and effective care is achieved and an effective learning environment is maintained
- Prioritize work to accommodate support of students
  (NMC, 2008)

CHAPTER 4

The aim of Chapter 4 is to explore the practice assessment document and the meaning of learning outcomes in more depth. There is a discussion on the role of the practice assessment document in the student's learning experience.

The chapter provides many practical exercises designed to help you understand the meaning of learning outcomes and plan learning experiences accordingly.

Box P.3 Mapping Chapter 4 to the NMC standards

- Use knowledge of the student's stage of learning to select appropriate learning opportunities to meet individual needs.
- Demonstrate a breadth of understanding of assessment strategies and ability to contribute to the total assessment process as part of the teaching team
- Initiate and respond to practice developments to ensure safe and effective care is achieved and an effective learning environment is maintained
- Be an advocate for students to support them accessing learning opportunities that meet their individual needs, involving a range of other professionals, patients, clients and carers
  (NMC, 2008)

CHAPTER 5

The aim of Chapter 5 is to investigate the process and purpose of the initial interview. Throughout the chapter you will be able to identify the main features, purpose and processes that should be considered when conducting an initial interview. You will also be able to improve your understanding of planning learning experiences that cater for a wide variety of student learning styles. In addition you will have an opportunity to explore ways to plan effectively for the initial interview event.

Box P.4 Mapping Chapter 5 to the NMC standards

- Use knowledge of the student's stage of learning to select appropriate learning opportunities to meet individual needs
- Facilitate the selection of appropriate learning strategies to integrate learning from practice and academic experiences
- Support students in identifying both learning needs and experience that are appropriate to their level of learning
- Identify aspects of the learning environment that could be enhanced, negotiating with others to make appropriate changes
- Contribute to the development of an environment in which effective practice is fostered, implemented, evaluated and disseminated
- Plan a series of learning experiences that will meet students' defined learning needs
- Be an advocate for students to support them accessing learning opportunities that meet their individual needs, involving a range of other professionals, patients, clients and carers
- Support students in applying an evidence base to their own practice

(NMC, 2008)

CHAPTER 6

The aim of Chapter 6 is to assist you in understanding the role of feedback in relation to the assessment process and the student learning experience. You will have the opportunity to identify the key aspects of verbal and written feedback and understand the relevance of the feedback sandwich in facilitating feedback. You will be required to consider your own professional accountability and responsibility in delivering feedback. By reading the chapter you will be able to identify areas where you may need to develop your own competence and confidence for feedback experiences.

Box P.5 Mapping Chapter 6 to the NMC standards

- Support students in critically reflecting upon their learning experiences in order to enhance future learning
- Foster professional growth, personal development and accountability through student support in practice
- Demonstrate a breadth of understanding of assessment strategies and ability to contribute to the total assessment process as part of the teaching team
- Provide constructive feedback to students and assist them in identifying future learning needs and actions, manage failing students so that they may enhance their performance and capabilities for safe and effective practice or be able to understand their failure and the implications of this for their future
- Contribute to evaluation of student learning and assessment experiences, proposing aspects for change resulting from such evaluation
- Support students in identifying both learning needs and experience that are appropriate to their level of learning
- Set and maintain professional boundaries that are sufficiently flexible for providing inter-professional care
  (NMC, 2008)

CHAPTER 7

The aim of Chapter 7 is to investigate the nature and function of the midpoint interview. There is an explanation of the purpose of the midpoint interview and a discussion on the essential components of a successful midpoint interview. Strategies for successfully conducting a midpoint interview are also addressed.

Box P.6 Mapping Chapter 7 to the NMC standards

- Use knowledge of the student's stage of learning to select appropriate learning opportunities to meet individual needs
- Support students in critically reflecting upon their learning experiences in order to enhance future learning

- Foster professional growth, personal development and accountability through student support in practice
- Demonstrate a breadth of understanding of assessment strategies and ability to contribute to the total assessment process as part of the teaching team
- Provide constructive feedback to students and assist them in identifying future learning needs and actions, manage failing students so that they may enhance their performance and capabilities for safe and effective practice or be able to understand their failure and the implications of this for their future
- Contribute to evaluation of student learning and assessment experiences, proposing aspects for change resulting from such evaluation
- Support students in identifying both learning needs and experience that are appropriate to their level of learning
- Set and maintain professional boundaries that are sufficiently flexible for providing inter-professional care
(NMC, 2008)

CHAPTER 8

The aim of Chapter 8 is to help you develop skills for managing a student who is not meeting the required level of competence on a placement. The chapter provides insight into identifying the early warning signs of failing students and also understanding the importance of accessing help and support for failing students early in the placement. By reading the chapter you will gain skills in planning effectively for how to fail a student when the situation arises.

Box P.7 Mapping Chapter 8 to the NMC standards

- Support students in critically reflecting upon their learning experiences in order to enhance future learning
- Provide constructive feedback to students and assist them in identifying future learning needs and actions, manage failing students so that they may enhance their performance and capabilities for safe and effective practice or be able to understand their failure and the implications of this for their future

Continued

Box P.7 Mapping Chapter 8 to the NMC standards—Cont'd

- Be accountable for confirming that students have met or not met the NMC competencies in practice and as a sign-off mentor confirm that students have met or not met the NMC standards of proficiency and are capable of safe and effective practice
- Provide feedback about the effectiveness of learning and assessing in practice
  (NMC, 2008)

CHAPTER 9

The aim of Chapter 9 is to explore the nature and function of the final interview. It includes a complete explanation regarding the purpose and importance of the final interview. You will have an opportunity to identify the essential components of a successful final interview and how to successfully conduct a final interview.

Box P.8 Mapping Chapter 9 to the NMC standards

- Support students in critically reflecting upon their learning experiences in order to enhance future learning
- Provide constructive feedback to students and assist them in identifying future learning needs and actions, manage failing students so that they may enhance their performance and capabilities for safe and effective practice or be able to understand their failure and the implications of this for their future
- Be accountable for confirming that students have met or not met the NMC competencies in practice and as a sign-off mentor confirm that students have met or not met the NMC standards of proficiency and are capable of safe and effective practice
- Provide feedback about the effectiveness of learning and assessing in practice
- Act as a resource to facilitate personal and professional development of others
  (NMC, 2008)

CHAPTER 10

The aim of this chapter is to gain an understanding of the role of the sign-off mentor. There will be the opportunity to explore the criteria for becoming a sign-off mentor and clarify the accountability of the sign-off mentor to the NMC when making the final assessment decision. In reading this chapter you will be able to appreciate the role of the ongoing achievement record in assisting the sign-off mentor to make their confirmation of a student's proficiency at the end of their programme.

Box P.9 Mapping Chapter 10 to the NMC standards

- Provide constructive feedback to students and assist them in identifying future learning needs and actions, manage failing students so that they may enhance their performance and capabilities for safe and effective practice or be able to understand their failure and the implications of this for their future
- Be accountable for confirming that students have met or not met the NMC competencies in practice and as a sign-off mentor confirm that students have met or not met the NMC standards of proficiency and are capable of safe and effective practice
- Provide feedback about the effectiveness of learning and assessing in practice
- Act as a resource to facilitate personal and professional development of others
- Participate in self and peer evaluation to facilitate personal development and contribute to the development of others
(NMC, 2008)

CHAPTER 11

The aim of Chapter 11 is to discuss and evaluate the mentor's role in relation to supporting students with a disability. The chapter provides an opportunity for discussing the definition of disability and how disabled students may best be supported on practice placements. The role of the mentor in supporting students and ensuring that reasonable adjustments are made is a key theme within this chapter.

> **Box P.10 Mapping Chapter 11 to the NMC standards**
>
> - Plan a series of learning experiences that will meet students' defined learning needs
> - Be an advocate for students to support them in accessing learning opportunities that meet their individual needs, involving a range of other professionals, patients, clients and carers
> - Prioritize work to accommodate support of students
> - Provide feedback about the effectiveness of learning and assessing in practice
>   (NMC, 2008)

CHAPTER 12

The aim of Chapter 12 is to explore the different types of challenging issues and situations that you may encounter as a mentor. Not only is there an opportunity to identify mentoring challenges in your clinical learning environment, you will be encouraged to reflect on how you manage challenges and identify practical measures to address challenges without compromising the assessment of student learning.

> **Box P.11 Mapping Chapter 12 to the NMC standards**
>
> - Identify and apply research and evidence-based practice to their area of practice
> - Contribute to strategies to increase or review the evidence base used to support practices
> - Support students in applying an evidence base to their own practice
> - Plan a series of learning experiences that will meet students' defined learning needs
> - Prioritize work to accommodate support of students
>   (NMC, 2008)

CHAPTER 13

The aim of Chapter 13 is to gain insight into the use of simulation in pre-registration nurse education. The chapter presents the key elements of simulated learning environments/simulation and how to evaluate strengths and weaknesses of your own teaching style in relation to facilitating simulation. There are tips and strategies presented that will assist you to plan effectively for a simulation session and for debriefing following simulation.

Box P.12 Mapping Chapter 13 to the NMC standards

- Support students in identifying both learning needs and experience that are appropriate to their level of learning
- Use a range of learning experiences involving patients, clients, carers and the professional team to meet defined learning needs
- Identify aspects of the learning environment that could be enhanced, negotiating with others to make appropriate changes
- Act as a resource to facilitate personal and professional development of others
  (NMC, 2008)

CHAPTER 14

The purpose of Chapter 14 is to explore strategies for evaluating the quality of the learning experience for students. The chapter outlines and examines why evaluation is a vitally important aspect of the mentoring role. By reading the chapter you will be able to identify strategies for evaluating the student experience in practice and also identify your own strengths and weaknesses as a mentor.

Box P.13 Mapping Chapter 14 to the NMC standards

- Identify and apply research and evidence-based practice to their area of practice
- Contribute to strategies to increase or review the evidence base used to support practices
- Contribute to evaluation of student learning and assessment experiences, proposing aspects for change resulting from such evaluation
- Participate in self and peer evaluation to facilitate personal development and contribute to the development of others
  (NMC, 2008)

FINAL WORDS

The authors would like to take this opportunity to thank each and every mentor who reads this book. As nurse educators with expert knowledge of the current demands and challenges in practice, we salute you. We understand how much time, dedication and personal effort goes into facilitating learning experiences of pre-registration students. We understand the difficulties and challenges of balancing the needs of students with the demands of patient care, and we acknowledge that very often your own time is given to ensure students receive support during their learning experience. We recognize that sometimes difficult decisions need to be made, and that thanks is not always given for your effort. As a group, we thank you. We hope that this book will be of support to you, as you facilitate and assess those who will become the future of our profession.

London, 2010   Karen Elcock
                                               Kath Sharples

Reference

Nursing and Midwifery Council (2008) *Standards to Support Learning and Assessment in Practice: NMC standards for mentors, practice teachers and teachers.* Nursing and Midwifery Council, London, available from www.nmc-uk.org

ACKNOWLEDGEMENTS

Thanks must be given to our colleagues from the Mentor Development Group and Disability and Widening Access Group who work tirelessly in developing strategies for supporting mentors and have influenced the content of this book.

In addition thanks are extended to Lindsay Towers, Disability Advisor at Thames Valley University, for sharing her expertise for the chapter on supporting students with disabilities.

Kath Sharples would like to thank all mentors at the North West London Hospitals NHS Trust who have contributed their wealth of experience and knowledge in supporting the pre-registration students of Thames Valley University. Your tireless efforts are a constant source of inspiration.

Special thanks to Ann for your love, endless encouragement, and wonderful cups of Earl Grey tea.

CHAPTER 1

MENTORING TODAY

Chapter Aims

The purpose of this chapter is to gain insight into the student's experience of mentorship. After reading this chapter you will be able to:

- Reflect on your own experiences of mentorship.
- Discuss the difference that mentorship can make to the placement learning experience for students.
- Identify the benefits of mentorship in terms of professional development and recruitment.

MENTORING AND NURSING

Having the opportunity to mentor a pre-registration nursing student is one of the most exciting and gratifying aspects of the nursing role. The benefits that can be gained from facilitating and developing the learning of others also provide intrinsic rewards that are unique within our profession. The prospect of being able to supervise, develop and make a lasting contribution to the learning needs of a pre-registration student should be valued as a key and fundamental aspect of your professional standing and career development.

YOUR EXPERIENCE AS A STUDENT

Every qualified nurse has a very unique advantage as they begin their mentoring journey. You will have the advantage of personal, first-hand experience of the mentoring role, as you were once a student yourself (see Activity 1.1). At key stages within your education as a nurse you will have been supervised and perhaps assessed by a mentor. No doubt you will have worked alongside and learnt from many mentors during your training, many of these will have made a valuable contribution to your eventual qualification and a lasting impression on your overall learning experience.

Activity 1.1 My experience as a student

Take some time to reflect back on your experience as a student nurse. Have a think about the mentors that you met during your nurse education programme. Consider the experiences that you would regard as positive, perhaps in terms of how the learning experience was facilitated, or the influence they may have had on your development. What attributes did you value in these mentors? You might like to make some brief notes on the factors that you valued most in your mentors.

Most of us would agree that during our nurse education we had the privilege of being mentored by a nurse whose care, skill and enthusiasm for their role as a mentor greatly contributed to a valuable learning experience as in Case study 1.1. Perhaps the mentor took time to understand your particular learning needs and then arranged for a broad range of experiences during your practice placement. Perhaps the mentor gave motivating and highly constructive feedback that enabled you to learn and develop additional knowledge and skills.

KEY POINT

Mentors who create a positive impression on students are also role-modelling positive attributes of the mentoring role for that student to demonstrate as a qualified nurse.

Case study 1.1 *A qualified nurse speaks of her experience as a student*

'I often think back to a mentor that I had during my first ever practice placement. She made such a difference. I was very nervous and scared because obviously everything was new, and she just always managed to say the right thing so that I didn't lose confidence. It was a very busy ward but every so often at the end of a shift she would say "let's have a cup of tea" and then we would sit there and talk about the day and how I felt. I realize now that she was doing a debrief – maybe something had happened that day that was difficult, like seeing someone in pain, and she just knew that I should be given the chance to talk and say how I felt. When I did my mentor course we were asked to talk about a mentor who made a difference to us. I thought of her straight away, and for the first time really appreciated what she had done. I decided then and there that she had not only been a great mentor herself, she had also shown me what sort of mentor I wanted to be.'

A mentor not only makes a valuable contribution to your learning, but also provides you with a benchmark for the type of mentor you should be aiming to become. As a student, you were not only learning to be a nurse, you were also learning the attributes of a 'good mentor'. This means that every time you mentor a student you are role-modelling how to be a mentor, not only by what you say or do, but by your general enthusiasm for the role. Now try Activity 1.2.

Activity 1.2 My experience as a student

Once again, take some time to reflect back on your experience as a student nurse. Have a think about the mentors that you met during your nurse education programme. Consider the experiences that you would regard as negative, perhaps in terms of how the learning experience was facilitated, or the influence they may have had on your development. What attributes gave you cause for concern or anxiety in these mentors? You might like to make some brief notes on the factors that made the experience negative or unrewarding.

For this reason it is almost impossible to understand why mentors do not always value and contribute to student learning with care and consideration. With first-hand knowledge of unhappy or discouraging experiences of mentoring as a student, all qualified nurses should have a clear understanding of how not to be. Mentors who fail to engage with students, possibly treating them as a nuisance can never justify this reaction, as they themselves were once a vulnerable and nervous learner themselves (see Case study 1.2).

KNOWING HOW IT FEELS

As a qualified nurse you know what it feels like to be a student. You know what it feels like to be nervous about your practice placement and who you will meet, and what will be expected of you. Yet for many nurses, the experiences as a student seem to be forgotten once qualification is achieved. The importance of good mentorship seems to be forgotten and replaced with aspirations of perceived dynamic post-registration modules of study. Mentorship modules can be viewed by nurses as a means to an end and are often the first course to be undertaken after qualifying. Yet we would argue that mentorship is not just a professional obligation, it is a professional privilege.

Case study 1.2 *A student speaks of her experience of a mentor*

'When I first meet my mentor on my practice placement I can usually tell if I'm wanted or not. It's only a first impression but I've realized that first impressions can tell you so much. I've learnt that mentors who smile and look me in the eye are the ones who will be supportive and thorough during the placement. The ones who look at you and can't even smile, well you just feel miserable; you're obviously not wanted and the placement will just be a struggle. I know it's busy and nurses have very little time, but how long does it take to smile? Those are the placements that you just try and get through, you know you won't enjoy it but what option do you have? You just grit your teeth and cross your fingers and hope the time passes as soon as possible. Sometimes you think to yourself "I only have to last 6 weeks and then I never have to meet these people again". I know that's not the best attitude but then again, it's sometimes all you can do.'

MENTORSHIP AND PROFESSIONAL DEVELOPMENT

In many ways the role of a mentor provides nurses with an extraordinary opportunity to develop professionally. Not only will you be directly involved in facilitating learning and assessment, but you will also be challenged to consider your own evidence base and standards of practice. During the course of your mentoring role you will have the opportunity to plan learning experiences, conduct interviews and meetings, provide formal and informal feedback, document clear reports, liaise with colleagues in the multidisciplinary team, make complex decisions and share your wealth of knowledge, skill and professionalism with someone who will truly value your experience. While developing these skills as part of your mentoring role will be rewarding in itself, you will also be developing a wealth of transferable skills that will enhance your future career opportunities.

MENTORING FOR THE RIGHT REASONS

It should be clear that being a mentor is a valuable role that will make a major difference not only to your own career, but also to the development of future professionals. As a mentor, students will be looking to you as a role model, a support person and a coach who will help them to navigate learning opportunities on practice placements. Students will be depending on you, and in your role as a mentor you really will be making a difference.

You cannot afford to take this role lightly or without preparation. If you treat your mentor role as insignificant then you will still be making a difference, but for all the wrong reasons. You should be very clear in your own mind then that being a mentor requires the same regard, respect and professionalism as you would give to all other aspects of your nursing role.

KEY POINT

If you do not value your mentor role then don't expect your student to value you. Apathy will breed apathy, enthusiasm will breed enthusiasm.

MENTORING AND RECRUITMENT

You may never have considered mentorship to be related to recruitment; however, it is one of the most powerful tools you have to attract job applications for your practice area. Students who spend their placement time with you will have an opportunity of comparing your placement with others during their programme. If they feel supported and valued as a student they will be encouraged to apply for a post as a newly qualified nurse. If they felt wanted and supported as a student then they will see this as evidence that they will also be supported during their early months as a qualified nurse. If your placement area has a reputation for being unsupportive of students you may well find it is not a favoured first post destination by newly qualified nurses.

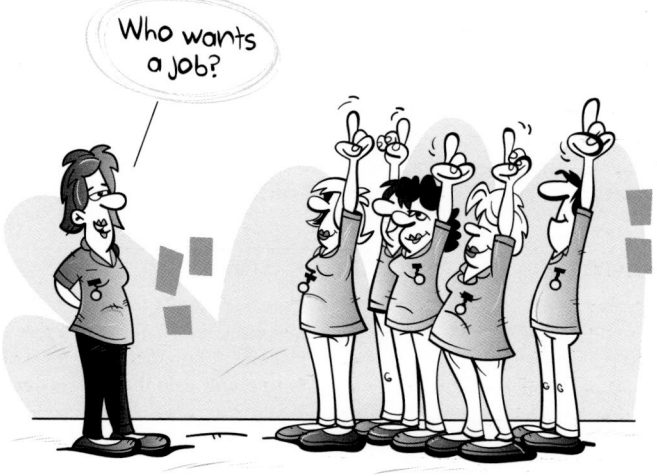

KEY POINT

Newly qualified nurses are very unlikely to apply for posts to areas where they have doubts about the support they will be given on their preceptorship programme. Supportive mentorship is a great opportunity to attract applications from former students.

MENTORING FOR SUCCESS

Throughout this book there will be the opportunity to explore all facets of the mentoring experience. The mentoring process will be covered as will the challenges of mentoring and professional requirements. However, any value that could be gained from these themes will be pointless unless you are committed to, and value mentoring as a part of your profession. Whatever highs your career brings, don't ever forget that you were once a student. Aim for excellence, and be the kind of mentor that your student is hoping you will be.

TOP TIPS

- If you want to be a great mentor then don't ever forget what it was like to be a student.
- Use your role as a mentor to develop transferable professional skills.
- Sell your practice area to students, demonstrate that you are supportive of learners and value the contribution they make to your team.
- Invite students to apply for posts in your practice area once qualified.

CHAPTER 2

MENTORING AND THE NMC

Chapter Aims

The purpose of this chapter is to gain an understanding of the *Standards to Support Learning and Assessment in Practice* set by the NMC for mentorship. After reading this chapter you will be able to:

- Identify the key points relating to mentorship in the NMC's Standards.
- Undertake a self-assessment of your knowledge, skills and competence against the NMC's developmental framework for mentors and develop an action plan to address any deficiencies.
- Develop a portfolio of evidence to demonstrate you meet the NMC's standards for mentors.

THE NMC STANDARDS FOR LEARNING AND ASSESSMENT IN PRACTICE

The NMC published their *Standards to Support Learning and Assessment in Practice* in August 2006 which became mandatory in September 2007. This means that all mentors must meet the requirements set out in these standards in order to support and assess students on programmes which lead to registration or a recordable qualification on the NMC register. It should be noted that the NMC republished the standards again in July 2008 with some minor amendments. The main changes were the addition of annexes, which were copies of circulars sent out by the NMC between 2006 and 2008, clarifying areas which had caused confusion or concern for mentors, placement providers and universities about:

- specialist practice qualifications
- the Practice Teacher standard
- applying due regard
- sign-off mentors and/or practice teachers
- guidance for small-scale service providers in relation to the standards
- the ongoing achievement record.

The 2008 standards were also updated to reflect wider policy changes, for example around equality and diversity. These standards can be downloaded from the NMC website www.nmc-uk.org and you are strongly recommended to download a copy if you are a mentor or about to become one.

The standards are set by the NMC in consultation with nurses, midwives, employers, the public and universities and are reviewed every five years. At the time that these standards were being reviewed, the NMC was also consulting on fitness to practice at the point of registration. Both consultations highlighted concerns about the quality of the support students receive in practice and led to a set of standards that are far more prescriptive than we have seen before and have specific requirements for mentors, practice teachers and teachers. While this chapter will focus on the NMC's requirements relating to mentors, you can read more about the requirements for practice teachers and teachers by reading the standards.

KEY POINT

The NMC's main purpose is to safeguard the health and wellbeing of the public. These standards reflect the need to ensure that students are capable of safe and effective practice at the point of registration.

WHAT ARE THE STANDARDS?

The standards describe a single developmental framework for mentors, practice teachers and teachers with outcomes for each role. The outcomes are grouped under eight domains for each stage:
1. Establishing effective working relationships.
2. Facilitation of learning.
3. Assessment and accountability.
4. Evaluation of learning.
5. Create an environment for learning.
6. Context of practice.
7. Evidence-based practice.
8. Leadership.

Each of the domains is underpinned by five principles that you can view in Box 2.1.

There are four stages to the framework and you can enter or exit the framework at any stage, you do not have to achieve one stage to get to the next (apart from stage one which applies to all registered nurses and midwives prior to entering stages 2, 3 or 4). The NMC expects that the majority of nurses and midwives will become a mentor (stage two) and

Box 2.1 Underpinning principles for the NMC developmental framework

The underpinning principles for supporting learning and assessment in practice for any student undertaking an NMC approved programme leading to registration or a qualification that is recordable on the register are that nurses and midwives who make judgements about whether a student has achieved the required standards of proficiency for safe and effective practice must:

(a) be on the same part or sub-part of the register as that which the student is intending to enter;

(b) have developed their own knowledge, skills and competency beyond that of registration through CPD – either formal or experiential learning – as appropriate to their support role;

(c) hold professional qualifications at an appropriate level to support and assess the students they mentor/teach, i.e. professional qualifications equal to, or at a higher level than, the students they are supporting and assessing and;

(d) have been prepared for their role to support and assess learning and met NMC defined outcomes. Also, that such outcomes have been achieved in practice and, where relevant, in academic settings, including abilities to support interprofessional learning. In addition:

(e) Nurses and midwives who have completed an NMC approved teacher preparation programme may record their qualification on the NMC register. Other teaching qualifications may be assessed against the NMC teacher outcomes through the NMC accreditation route.

(NMC, 2008, p16)

it is likely that most will stop there. Each of the four stages is outlined in Table 2.1.

In addition to the developmental framework the NMC standards also introduced some new requirements which we will also look at in this chapter:

- how to become a mentor
- the local register of mentors
- sign-off mentors
- due regard.

Table 2.1 The four stages in the developmental framework			
Stage	**Role**	**Required if you wish to:**	**Where recorded**
One	Nurse or Midwife	Facilitate students and others to develop their competence	N/A
Two	Mentor	Support and assess pre-registration nursing/midwifery students	Local Register of Mentors
Three	Practice Teacher	Support and assess specialist community public health students	Local Register of Practice Teachers
Four	Teacher	Be based in Higher Education and support learning and assessment of students on NMC approved programmes and often a prerequisite for lecturer practitioner/practice educator roles	NMC Register (requires a fee)

BECOMING A MENTOR

In order to become a mentor you need to meet the requirements set out in the standards. This can be achieved in a number of ways depending on whether you already hold a mentor qualification or are about to set out on the path to become a mentor.

Since September 2007 the only route to becoming a mentor is by undertaking an NMC-approved mentor preparation programme delivered by a university. While each university is likely to call their programme by a different name it has to meet specific standards set by the NMC and it has to be approved by the NMC as meeting those standards. Before becoming a mentor you have to have been registered for at least one year. Figure 2.1 is a flow diagram that may help you to determine whether you are a mentor or not.

IF YOU ALREADY HAVE A MENTOR QUALIFICATION

Mentors who have completed a previously recognized mentorship programme prior to September 2007 can still be mentors as long as they are on the mentor register. Examples of courses which are usually recognized are:

- ENB 997 or 998
- a mentorship course run at your university between April 2002 and August 2007

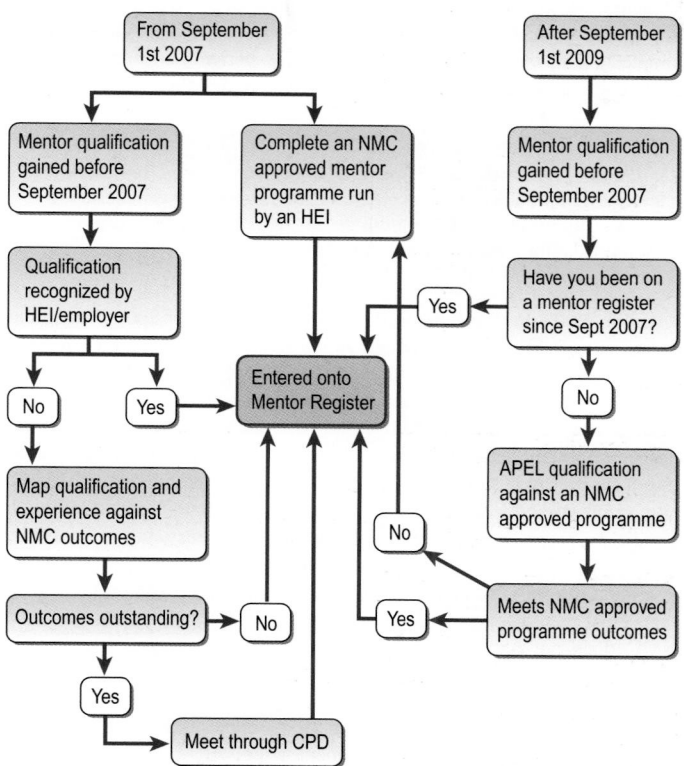

Figure 2.1 How to become a mentor

- City and Guilds 730/7307
- Certificate in Education
- BSc Specialist Practitioner where teaching and assessing was also included.

If none of the above applies to you and you have been acting as a mentor then the NMC advises that you should map your qualification and experience against the current mentor standards and identify if there are any outcomes that your qualification (or the experience you have had as a mentor) have not met. These deficiencies need to be met through continuing professional development. See the end of this chapter for a simple tool to map your qualification and experience against with suggested activities you can undertake to meet any deficiencies.

KEY POINT

If you can't remember which mentorship course you attended check the information provided on the certificate you received on completion. If you are still unsure regarding your status then discuss the course you completed with a lecturer from the university.

In July 2009 the NMC advised that after 1 September 2009 if you hold one of the qualifications listed above but have not yet been on a mentor register then you must either undertake an NMC approved mentor preparation programme or demonstrate that you have met the outcomes through the Accreditation of Prior and (Experiential) Learning (AP(E)L) process at a university. This only applies if you have never been entered into a register (e.g. you may have taken a break from nursing or worked abroad or worked in an area that did not take students) and so although you held a mentor qualification you had not been practising as a mentor.

Once you have successfully completed your mentorship programme you must inform your employer so that they can place you on their local register of mentors. At this point you are allowed to mentor students. The NMC does not require you to inform them as it is your employer's responsibility to hold the register of mentors not the NMCs.

Nurses who are on Part 2 of the NMC register (formerly called Enrolled Nurses) can act as a mentor to a student as long as they have a mentor qualification and are on a mentor register.

THE LOCAL MENTOR REGISTER

In order to be a mentor you must be entered onto a local register of mentors. It is the responsibility of the placement provider to set up and maintain this register unless they are what the NMC refer to as a small placement provider. A small placement provider would be somewhere like a nursing home or a small independent hospital. In these cases it is the responsibility of the university to maintain the register of mentors. The NMC does not state what information should be kept on the register; however, in Table 2.2 are some of the headings that may be used to

Table 2.2 Suggested headings for the local register of mentors	
Headings in Register	**Why needed**
The mentor's name	
Professional qualification(s)	To ensure due regard is applied
Mentorship qualification and when obtained	Proof you have met NMC requirements to be entered onto the register
Date of last mentor update	All mentors are required by the NMC to update annually
Whether a sign-off mentor	Mentors who are also sign-off mentors must be annotated on the register
Date of last triennial review	All mentors are required to be reviewed every three years to ensure that they continue to meet the NMC's requirements

compile a local register of mentors and the reasons why they are needed. Don't worry about due regard and sign-off mentors as we will look at these later in the chapter.

The reason for a mentor register is to allow both the placement provider and the university to reassure themselves that there are sufficient mentors who meet the NMC requirements as set out in the standards to support the students being placed within each practice placement. The register is shared with the university at least twice a year.

STAYING ON THE LIVE REGISTER OF MENTORS

Once on the register you become what the NMC refers to as a *live mentor*. However, in order to stay a live mentor and therefore remain on the mentor register you are required to meet certain criteria which are:
- to update annually
- to mentor at least two students over a three-year period
- to participate in a triennial review to demonstrate that you continue to meet the NMC's requirements as set out in the standards.

You have a responsibility to ensure that the person who holds the local register of mentors where you work is kept informed of the following:
- when you attend updates
- what type of update you attended
- any changes that may impact on your role (e.g. taking maternity leave, changing your place of work within the organization) so that they can update the register accordingly.

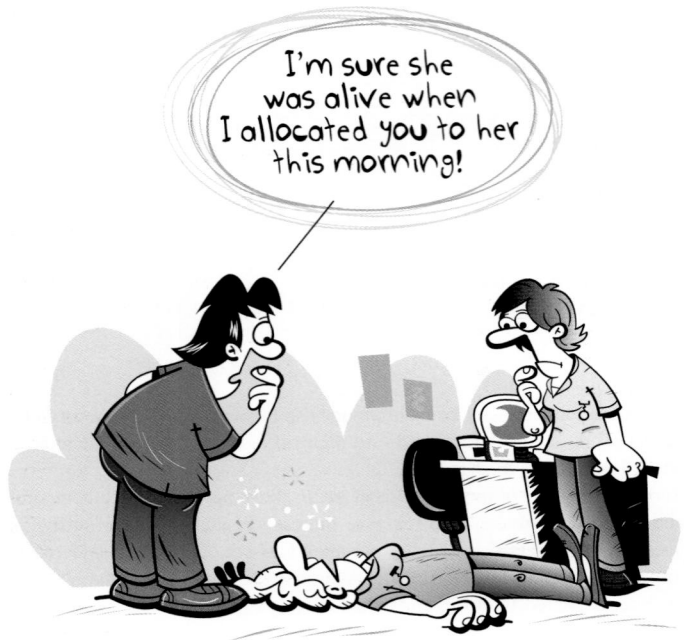

MENTOR UPDATING

The NMC requires all mentors to update annually. The aim of annual updating is to ensure that mentors and practice teachers continue to:

- have current knowledge of NMC approved programmes
- understand the implications of changes to NMC requirements
- understand issues relating to supporting students
- make valid and reliable assessments of competence and fitness for safe and effective practice (NMC, 2008 p. 9).

You can think of updating like a car MOT (motor vehicle test), which has to be carried out on your car each year. If you update as a mentor in January then you must ensure you update in January each year. For example, when your car fails its MOT you are no longer allowed to drive it until you have remedied any deficiencies found. Similarly, if you fail to update yourself as a mentor annually then you can no longer be considered a live mentor and may not mentor students until you have updated again. The person who holds the local live register of mentors is required to remove you from the mentor register until they have been informed that you have updated.

As you can see the NMC treats mentor updating very seriously and they will seek assurance that the register is kept up-to-date as part of the regular quality monitoring that takes place of all NMC approved nursing and midwifery programmes.

Keeping yourself updated can be a challenge and many mentors say they find it difficult to attend annual updates. The NMC doesn't specify what counts as an update but states that it '*must include the opportunity to meet and explore assessment and supervision issues with other mentors/practice teachers*' and to have '*explored as a group the validity and reliability of judgements made when assessing practice in challenging circumstances.*' (NMC, 2008 p.12).

In a guidance document published on their website in February 2009 the NMC added in the requirement that mentors should have the opportunity to meet up with other mentors face-to-face suggesting a slightly more formal approach to updating. They also recommend that an update can be achieved in a variety of ways but indicate that it should be ongoing throughout the year and supported by a range of other activities, some of which are explored below (see also Case study 2.1).

THE FORMAL MENTOR UPDATE

Formal mentor updates are usually run by your local university, often in partnership with the NHS Trusts/organizations with which it links at a central location. They may be anything from one hour to a whole day and ideally will include an opportunity for the mentors attending to discuss issues around supporting and assessing students, including supporting the challenging student. Formal updates tend to be planned in advance, allowing you to book into them and may be linked to your other mandatory updating sessions that your employer is required to run, such as moving and handling, equality and diversity, etc. The formal update tends to be the preferred option by the NMC as it offers the face-to-face approach and the opportunity to have a discussion around assessment and supervision with other mentors/practice teachers. However, a formal mentor update could also be held just for you or you and your colleagues in your ward/department/unit by the lecturer from your local university.

A MENTOR CONFERENCE

This is usually run by the local university and is usually a whole day event covering issues around supporting and assessing students and may also include other healthcare professional groups.

COMPLETION OF A MENTOR WORKBOOK/ON-LINE UPDATE

This may be a hard copy booklet that you work through or it may be completed on-line via your university website or your employer's website. This is a popular approach for staff who may find it difficult to attend a formal update or conference. The disadvantage of this style of update is that it does not offer the opportunity for you to discuss issues around supporting and assessing students with colleagues. However, you could complete the workbook in conjunction with colleagues either working through the workbook/on-line programme together or discussing your answers after completion, perhaps with a lecturer from your university who visits your area.

READING MENTORSHIP ARTICLES

A number of nursing journals regularly publish articles on mentorship and often these will have a series of activities for you to undertake while reading through them. They may even offer you the opportunity to gain a certificate of learning for completing a small piece of work on completion of the article. If you choose this method to update yourself remember to keep a copy of the work you undertake in your portfolio as evidence of learning and updating. Again learning will be enhanced if you do this with other colleagues so encouraging discussion of the issues raised in the article(s).

DROP-IN GROUPS OR MENTOR SURGERIES

These are usually held in larger placement provider organizations by the local university and/or staff with a responsibility for mentorship in your organization. They are usually held on a regular basis throughout the year and offer mentors (and usually students) an opportunity to drop in and discuss issues arising around placement learning and assessment. This approach meets the NMC's requirements around opportunities to discuss supervision and assessment issues.

PARTICIPATION IN OSCES

OSCEs are Objective Structured Clinical Examinations. They usually comprise simulated learning events in a skills laboratory, which are assessed against agreed criteria. Universities run these as part of nursing and midwifery programmes and are always keen for mentors to participate in them so if interested contact your local university. In Chapter 13 we will cover simulated learning in far more detail.

Working with other mentors and academic colleagues in assessing students in a skills laboratory can be a useful way to update yourself on how students are being taught and gain further insight into the student curriculum. You will also have an excellent opportunity to discuss the assessment process and the grades to be given to the students being assessed. This method of updating also meets the NMC's requirement for an opportunity to discuss assessment of practice learning and in particular the challenges of ensuring the reliability and validity of assessments.

Other activities or resources that can be used to supplement the more formal updates or informal group discussions are:

- mentor newsletters
- shadowing
- reflective practice
- role play
- development of resources for students on placement

Case study 2.1 A mentor reflects on her mentor record

'All mentors in my Trust have been issued with a mentor record designed by the university. It has three sections where I can easily record information about mentor updates I've attended and also the students I've mentored during the year. Every year at annual appraisal my manager reviews my mentor record and confirms that I've kept myself up to date and meet the NMC standards to continue on the mentor register. It also helps me to keep track of when I need updating and consolidate anything that I don't know. In the last year I've been able to keep myself up to date by attending the mentor update held by a lecturer, read the mentor newsletter and also looked at some student assessment documents on the universities practice education website. I really enjoy being a mentor and keeping up to date makes the whole experience really easy.'

- participating or leading on educational audits of practice placements
- participating in curriculum development groups.

Whichever methods you use to update remember to record them in your portfolio with the dates and type of activities undertaken, together with any additional evidence you may have of updating as you will need this for your triennial review.

THE TRIENNIAL REVIEW AND MENTOR PORTFOLIO

All mentors are required to participate in a triennial review in order to demonstrate that they are continuing to meet the NMC's requirements for remaining on the local register of mentors. This may take place as part of your annual personal appraisal process or be a separate event; your employer can decide what is most effective for their organization. The NMC has stipulated the evidence you must have for your triennial review but there is additional information that you should also keep which we discuss below. The evidence the NMC requires is highlighted in Table 2.3.

YOUR MENTOR PORTFOLIO

The suggested contents are:
- Your name
- Professional qualifications (including field of practice)
- Title of the mentor preparation programme you attended, along with where studied and date passed
- Record of students mentored (i.e. type of student, dates mentored, stage of programme student on (first/second/third year))
- Reflections on experience of mentoring each student, how any challenges were addressed (optional)
- Record of mentor updates (date, type of update)
- Record of the opportunities you have had to meet and explore assessment and supervision issues with other mentors/practice teachers
- Record of participating in a group activity to explore the validity and reliability of judgements made when assessing practice in challenging circumstances
- Record of any other activities that relate to supporting learning and assessment in practice (e.g. participating in a curriculum development group, development of resources, literature reviews, etc.)
- Review of performance as a mentor as part of your annual professional appraisal (optional). This can be linked into the Knowledge and Skills

Table 2.3 Evidence required for triennial review	
Evidence required (NMC, 2008, p12)	**Rationale and suggested strategies for demonstrating evidence**
To have mentored at least two students (practice teachers to have supervised at least one student) with due regard (extenuating circumstances permitting) within the three-year period	In order to maintain your competence as a mentor you need to be using your skills mentoring students. For students to count they must be students from the same part of the register as you (due regard). You therefore need to keep a record of the dates you have mentored students over the last three years
Participated in annual updating – to include an opportunity to meet and explore assessment and supervision issues with other mentors/practice teachers	Annual updating is discussed in more detail below but you will need to record the dates you updated for the last three years and how you updated yourself. The second part of the sentence can be achieved by attending a formal update with other mentors where discussions took place or it could be a record of a more informal meeting with other mentors to explore issues in general or reflection with other mentors about a particular student or students you have mentored
Explored as a group activity the validity and reliability of judgements made when assessing practice in challenging circumstances	This could be part of a formal update with a scenario or discussing a real student (maintaining confidentiality) who posed a particular challenge. Keep a record of this activity in your portfolio
Mapped ongoing development in their role against the current NMC mentor/practice teacher standards	See Box 2.3
Been deemed to have met all requirements needed to be maintained on the local register as a mentor, sign-off mentor or practice teacher	See your mentor portfolio

Framework for Learning and Development (Core Dimension 2 – Personal & People Development)
- Completion of the mentor self-assessment tool at the end of this chapter with action plan
- Evidence of your three observed assessments to become a sign-off mentor if applicable
- A section for signing off your triennial review with your manager.

KEY POINT

A mentor record or mentor portfolio is a handy way of keeping track of what updates you have and haven't attended. Ask a lecturer at the university to see if one is already available for you to complete. If not, then consider developing your own record system.

WHEN IS MY TRIENNIAL REVIEW DUE?

Your triennial review will be due 3 years after you were placed on the mentor register and every 3 years after that. For mentors who were placed on the live register when the standards became mandatory in September 2007 this would mean they would be due in September 2010, then September 2013, September 2016, etc. For mentors who completed an NMC approved mentorship programme after September 2007 it would be 3 years after completing that programme.

APPLYING DUE REGARD

The concept of due regard was introduced by the NMC in their standards in 2006 and has been an area which has caused some confusion and challenges for mentors. By due regard the NMC means:

> *NMC registrants who make judgements about whether a student has achieved the required standards of proficiency for safe and effective practice must be on the same part or sub-part of the register as that which the student is intending to enter (NMC, 2008 p. 60).*

In order to understand due regard you will find it helpful to have an understanding of the different parts of the NMC register, as outlined in Box 2.2.

All nurses and midwives are required to register with the NMC in order to practice. The register has three parts:

1. Nursing.
2. Midwifery.
3. Specialist Community Public Health Nursing.

A nurse or midwife can also register as a Specialist Community Public Health Nurse if they have met the required entry standards for this part of the register.

Box 2.2 The parts of the NMC Register

Level 1 Nurses Sub-part 1	Level 2 Nurses Sub-part 2
Adult	Adult
Mental Health	Mental Health
Learning Disabilities	Learning Disabilities
Children	General
	Fever

Midwives' part of the Register

Midwifery

Specialist Community Public Health Nurses' part of the Register
Specialist Community Public Health Nursing – HV
Specialist Community Public Health Nursing – SN
Specialist Community Public Health Nursing – OH
Specialist Community Public Health Nursing – FHN
Specialist Community Public Health Nursing

Nursing has four fields of practice for level 1 nurses and five fields of practice for level 2 nurses and Specialist Community Public Health Nursing has five fields of practice.

To put it simply, due regard is all about ensuring that a mentor who is assessing a student's proficiency is from the same part of the register and the same field (commonly called branch in nursing) as their student. So for example the proficiencies for a student who intends to register as a mental health nurse can only be assessed by a nurse registered for the field of mental health (RNMH). Surprisingly a Health Visitor (Specialist Community Public Health Nurse HV) who spends the majority of their time working with children cannot assess a nursing student on a child branch programme unless they themselves are also registered on the nurse's part of the register and in the field of child health.

This does not mean that a nurse from a different part of the register or field cannot assess a student at all, but the student's placement has to be overseen by a mentor from the same part of the register and field of practice as the student (see Case study 2.2).

The same process applies where a student is placed with a person who has specific relevant specialist knowledge or the placement provides particular learning opportunities for the student, for example, in the criminal justice system for a mental health nurse, with a social worker for a learning disabilities student or on a gynaecology ward for a midwife.

Case Study 2.2 *Applying due regard*

Sarah is a child branch student who is on a 4-week placement in a Learning Disability unit in order to gain experience of caring for children with challenging behaviour. All the nursing staff on the unit are Learning Disability nurses so cannot assess Sarah with due regard. Sarah is allocated one of the Learning Disability nurses as her supervisor for the placement but her university has arranged for a mentor who is a children's nurse to oversee the placement. The mentor, the supervisor and Sarah meet at the start, mid-point and end of the placement. They agree the activities that Sarah will be focusing on during her placement in order to achieve the specific learning outcomes for that placement; with the mentor advising how these should be interpreted in the context of children's nursing. The supervisor can assess component skills specifically related to learning disability nursing but it is the mentor, in discussion with Sarah and the supervisor, who confirms whether Sarah has met the required overall proficiency at the end of the placement.

Due regard does not apply to:
- Student nurses in their first year who are not on a branch-specific placement
- Placements where the assessment is formative only.

> **KEY POINT**
>
> You can ensure your practice area meets due regard by forming a simple list of each mentor and writing next to it the part of the register they appear under. You may be surprised to find that some mentors in your practice placement belong to more than one part of the register.

THE SIGN-OFF MENTOR – A BRIEF INTRODUCTION

The sign-off mentor is a new role introduced by the NMC in their standards in 2006 which became mandatory for all students commencing a programme leading to registration from 1 September 2007.

A sign-off mentor is a registrant who:
- has met all the criteria to be a mentor and
- has met additional criteria to be a sign-off mentor and
- is annotated on the live register of mentors as a sign-off mentor.

All practice teachers and midwifery mentors are required to meet the requirements as a sign-off mentor through their mentor preparation programme. In other words all practice teachers and midwifery mentors have to be sign-off mentors.

Only a sign-off mentor can sign-off a student's practice proficiency at the end of their programme. For student nurses this means that the mentor on their final long placement must be a sign-off mentor who is on the same part and field of the NMC register as the student will be applying to. In Chapter 10 we will look at sign-off mentors in far more detail.

THE MENTOR'S ROLE AND RESPONSIBILITY

Your role and responsibilities as a mentor are wide ranging and should never be taken lightly. The key areas you are responsible and accountable for from the NMC's Standards (NMC, 2008 p. 19) include:

- Organizing and co-ordinating student learning activities in practice.
- Supervising students in learning situations and providing them with constructive feedback on their achievements.
- Setting and monitoring achievement of realistic learning objectives.
- Assessing total performance – including skills, attitudes and behaviours.
- Providing evidence as required by programme providers of student achievement or lack of achievement.
- Liaising with others (e.g. mentors, sign-off mentors, practice facilitators, practice teachers, personal tutors, programme leaders) to provide feedback, identify any concerns about the student's performance and agree action as appropriate.
- Providing evidence for, or acting as, sign-off mentors with regard to making decisions about achievement of proficiency at the end of a programme.

ASSESSING YOUR COMPETENCE

You should now be aware of what a mentor is and the criteria set by the NMC for taking on this responsibility. You will be aware of what options are available to you to keep yourself updated and 'live' on a mentor register. Take some time now to complete the self-assessment checklist in Box 2.3. By assessing yourself against the NMC standards you will be able to clearly ascertain your strengths as a mentor and areas that require further development. As you move through this book you will have the opportunity of addressing these areas further.

Box 2.3 Self-Assessment Form for Mentors based on the NMC Framework to Support Learning and Assessment in Practice (NMC, 2008)

Review each of the learning outcomes below against your mentor qualification and experience as a mentor. If you tick No for any outcomes, what actions will you take to remedy this deficit (some ideas are given)?

Outcomes for a Mentor

1. Establishing effective working relationships	Yes/no	Possible actions to take
Demonstrate an understanding of factors that influence how students integrate into practice settings.		Review or prepare an orientation pack for students.
Provide ongoing and constructive support to facilitate transition from one learning environment to another.		Discuss how to use the ongoing achievement record effectively with the link lecturer.
Have effective professional and interprofessional working relationships to support learning for entry to the register.		Identify IPL experiences available to students.

2. Facilitation of learning	Yes/no	Possible actions to take
Use knowledge of the student's stage of learning to select appropriate learning opportunities to meet individual needs.		Review course information from the HEI or relevant practice assessment documents and identify appropriate learning opportunities for each stage.
Facilitate the selection of appropriate learning strategies to integrate learning from practice and academic experiences.		
Support students in critically reflecting upon their learning experiences in order to enhance future learning.		Read up on reflective practice techniques.

THE MENTOR'S ROLE AND RESPONSIBILITY

	Yes/no	Possible actions to take
3. Assessment and accountability		**Possible actions to take**
Foster professional growth, personal development and accountability through student support in practice.		Read Kathleen Duffy's report on the NMC website or Review Practice Assessment documents or Sit in on assessment process with a Sign-off Mentor.
Demonstrate a breadth of understanding of assessment strategies and ability to contribute to the total assessment process as part of the teaching team.		
Provide constructive feedback to students and assist them in identifying future learning needs and actions, manage failing students so that they may enhance their performance and capabilities for safe and effective practice or be able to understand their failure and the implications of this for their future.		
Be accountable for confirming that students have met or not met the NMC competencies in practice and as a sign-off mentor confirm that students have met or not met the NMC standards of proficiency and are capable of safe and effective practice.		Review the section on sign-off mentors in the NMC's Standards for Learning and Assessment in Practice.
4. Evaluation of learning	**Yes/no**	**Possible actions to take**
Contribute to evaluation of student learning and assessment experiences, proposing aspects for change resulting from such evaluation.		Discuss student evaluations with your peers and/or Link Lecturer and plan strategies to improve or enhance the learning experience.
Participate in self and peer evaluation to facilitate personal development and contribute to the development of others.		Discuss with your manager at appraisal or Triennial Review.
5. Creating an environment for learning	**Yes/no**	**Possible actions to take**
Support students to identify both learning needs and experience that are appropriate to their level of learning.		Use information from your HEI about the students' programme to identify learning opportunities for your students.

Continued

Box 2.3 Self-Assessment Form for Mentors based on the NMC Framework to Support Learning and Assessment in Practice (NMC, 2008)—Cont'd

Use a range of learning experiences involving patients, clients, carers and the professional team to meet defined learning needs.		Use information from your HEI about the student's programme to identify learning opportunities for your students.
Identify aspects of the learning environment which could be enhanced, negotiating with others to make appropriate changes.		Review the student evaluations of your area for aspects to enhance.
Act as a resource to facilitate personal and professional development of others.		Co-mentor with a new mentor to develop their skills.
6. Context of practice	**Yes/no**	**Possible actions to take**
Contribute to the development of an environment in which effective practice is fostered, implemented, evaluated and disseminated.		
Set and maintain professional boundaries that are sufficiently flexible for providing inter-professional care.		Participate in clinical audit in your area, involve students where possible.
Initiate and respond to practice developments to ensure safe and effective care is achieved and an effective learning environment is maintained.		
7. Evidence-based practice	**Yes/no**	**Possible actions to take**
Identify and apply research and evidence based practice to their area of practice.		Set up a journal club. Review policies and procedures within your area. Review a key policy, e.g. National Standard Framework that is applicable to your area.
Contribute to strategies to increase or review the evidence base used to support practices.		
Support students in applying an evidence base to their own practice.		

8. Leadership

	Yes/no	Possible actions to take
Plan a series of learning experiences that will meet students defined learning needs		Look at relevant Module Study Guides & Practice assessment docs, Mentor Handbook, etc. to plan a series of learning experiences for students coming to your area.
Be an advocate for students to support them accessing learning opportunities that meet their individual needs, involving a range of other professionals, patients, clients and carers		
Prioritize work to accommodate support of students		
Provide feedback about the effectiveness of learning and assessing in practice		Participate in the educational audit of your area.

Evidence/Notes arising from self-assessment exercise:

_____

_____

_____

_____

Actions to be undertaken to ensure you meet NMC Competencies:

_____

_____

_____

Signed:

Date Actions Achieved:

TOP TIPS

- Find out what the agreed process is for mentor updating in your organization and set the date for your next update in your diary.
- Keep your portfolio up to date.
- Put the date for your next triennial review in your diary.

Reference

Nursing and Midwifery Council, 2008. *Standards to Support Learning and Assessment in Practice: NMC standards for mentors, practice teachers and teachers.* Nursing and Midwifery Council, London, available from www.nmc-uk.org.

CHAPTER 3

PREPARING FOR STUDENTS

Chapter Aims

The purpose of this chapter is to gain insight into the preparation that may be required prior to mentoring a student. After reading this chapter you will be able to:

- Identify the key elements of a learning environment.
- Evaluate strengths and weaknesses of your own student preparation.
- Plan effectively for a student's arrival.

BEFORE THE STUDENT ARRIVES

The fact that students spend 50% of their programme on practice placements can result in some areas having a constant flow of students through the door. For many mentors, having students in your practice area on a regular basis can end up feeling like it's part of the routine, especially if new students are arriving almost weekly. However, spare a thought for the student in all this. While you may tend to see them as 'just another student', they will arrive in your practice area with all the fears and anxieties that are entirely normal when entering a foreign environment. From the student's point of view, the first day of placement is vitally important. If a student feels welcomed straight away, this is the best possible start and they will be more likely to maintain a positive outlook throughout the entire placement. There is just no substitute for a student going home after the first day thinking 'I love my ward/unit/clinic/day centre'. However, if a student gets off to a bad start they will feel very let down, and even more anxious about the weeks to come.

STUDENT EXPECTATIONS

Every student that commences placement in your practice area will arrive with a certain set of expectations. These expectations will be based partly on previous experiences, partly on the information they may have received from other students and/or the university, and partly on any previous contact they may have had with your practice area. This may have been in the form of a pre-placement visit or by looking at on online profile of the placement. If a student's expectations are not met they may begin the placement with a negative mindset. On the other hand, meet these expectations and the placement can begin on a high note.

Likewise, you will also have expectations about the student. If your student meets these expectations on the first day this will no doubt influence your opinion regarding them. If they do not meet your expectations then no doubt you may feel let down and frustrated. Yet the expectations that students and mentors may have for each other may be based on unreasonable or unrealistic assumptions or misunderstandings that can only be resolved through honest and open communication. This type of communication must take place before the placement begins, and as such, is a vital part of pre-placement preparation. This means that before a student arrives in your practice area you will need to have prepared specifically for their arrival. You should not rely on the hope that everything will just magically fall into place; it will take planning, co-ordination and communication throughout your whole team.

In this chapter we will explore issues you should consider when preparing for a student's arrival, how to identify potential problems, and specific aspects of preparation such as information packs and off-duty considerations. It is only once these preparations are considered that you will be fully prepared for accepting students into your learning environment.

IS YOUR PRACTICE AREA PREPARED?

Let us assume that a student nurse is starting their placement in your practice area next week. Now stop and think for a moment. Would you be prepared? Before you consider the answer, have a look and reflect on the following two questions:

1. Is there any particular preparation that is routinely done by your clinical area before a student arrives?
2. Is there a system in place that ensures that the staff in your area are prepared for students' arrival?

TIME FOR HONESTY

If you have answered yes to both of these questions, then this is great, your practice area is well on the way to preparing for students. You will be able to use this chapter to identify ways that you may be able to develop and improve on your current practices. However, if you have

Case study 3.1 *A student speaks about her first day of placement*

'My worst experience was in my second year when I started a placement in a day-care clinic. I had already done a pre-placement visit the week before and met the manager who was lovely, so I turned up on my first day feeling really confident. It was just awful, because the manager was off sick and hadn't told anyone I was coming. The nurse in charge was new herself and was really rude. She said I must be in the wrong place because the manager had not said anything about expecting a student. I had to call the university to prove that I was meant to be there, and even then she didn't apologise. I just felt in the way the whole day, as if it was my fault that I had turned up when the manager was off-sick. No one knew who my mentor was meant to be and I was just told to wait until the manager returned the next day. It was just the worst day ever.'

answered no to either or both questions then the fact is that your area is not at all prepared for students.

Without specific preparatory systems in place the truth is that students will be faced with a 'lucky dip' of experiences on their first day. They may get lucky and have a positive experience and be welcomed, however they are just as likely to be ignored, forgotten or made to feel unwanted. Consider the scenario in Case study 3.1.

Quite obviously the events outlined in Case study 3.1 are just unacceptable, and from a mentor's perspective, highly unprofessional. However, without an identified plan, a student's first day can easily become a horrible experience for them. Sometimes it goes wrong due to unforeseen circumstances such as low staffing numbers due to sickness; however, often it reflects poor preparation or inexperienced mentors. Unfortunately this is a reality that is all too common, and while it is rarely the result of deliberate actions, this does little to rectify the situation. If a student's first experience of practice is of feeling unwanted and rejected, you will find yourself in the unhappy position of having to salvage the placement by re-establishing trust before you can move on.

WHAT CAN GO WRONG?

Crossing your fingers and hoping that the first day of a student's placement just works out is not the way to ensure a student has a satisfactory placement in your clinical area. You will need to accept therefore that quite a bit of planning and preparation needs to go into your clinical environment before a student arrives.

Obviously the best-case scenario in Activity 3.1 represents what would be the ideal first day for any student. However, the reality is that very often it is the opposite of this that actually takes place (see Activity 3.2).

Activity 3.1 Best-case scenario of a student's first day

Let's look at planning your clinical environment from the student's perspective. Imagine you are about to walk through the door on your first day of a new placement. What is the best-case scenario for what you would like to happen next? There are some ideas listed to get you started, however you might like to add in your own ideas based on your own experiences. As you were a student once too, you could even use this opportunity to reflect on your own experiences when you were training to be a nurse.

Best-case Scenario

- You are met by your mentor and welcomed by name – it is clear you are expected.
- Your mentor introduces you to the staff on duty that day.
- You are shown where you can store your bag/coat, etc.
- You are welcomed into the team working that day and encouraged to join in on handover/team meeting.

Activity 3.2 Worst-case scenario of a student's first day

Once again imagine you are about to walk through the door on your first day of a new placement. However, this time you are required to reflect on the following. What is the worst-case scenario for what might happen next? Just like Activity 3.1 there are suggestions to get you started and you are able to add in your own ideas based on your own experiences.

Worst-case Scenario

No-one greets you, no one can find your name on any list – it is clear that you are not expected.

No-one introduces you to anyone, and no-one seems to know who your mentor should be.

You are told that there is nowhere for students to put their belongings as all lockers and cupboards are full.

You sit in on handover/team meeting but feel as if you are in the way.

We must therefore identify what potential problems might occur, so systems can be put in place to prevent problems before they arise.

The best- and worst-case scenarios represent the two extremes of a student experience. No-one is expecting your clinical area to be perfect; however, as a mentor you should be striving to create a positive experience and enable students to feel welcomed on their first day. Without planning how to achieve this, the student is more than likely to experience elements of the worst-case scenario rather than the best-case scenario.

KEY POINT

When planning for a student's arrival, identify every element of what you would like to happen on the first day and then plan step by step what needs to be done to achieve that goal. Your list may look very similar to your list in the best-case scenario.

CREATING A LEARNING ENVIRONMENT

Before any student arrives in your clinical area you must ensure that you have prepared a learning environment that is suitable for them. Students are not just with you to complete a set amount of hours. The purpose of a practice placement is for students to learn while they are with you, through practising skills, increasing their knowledge and role modelling the professional behaviours of staff. It is your responsibility therefore to ensure that your area as a practice placement is a suitable environment for students to learn in and through.

LEARNING OPPORTUNITIES

Start by asking yourself these questions:
1. What opportunities are there for students to learn in my area?
2. What activities do we undertake that students might learn from and through?

No doubt you will be able to identify a number quite quickly. For example, drug rounds, wound dressings, patient assessment and observation, to name a few. The term used to describe these activities is *learning opportunities*. A learning opportunity is any event or activity that exists in a placement area that a student might learn something from either by taking part or observing. Now try Activity 3.3.

Activity 3.3 Learning Opportunities

Take some time to note down the learning opportunities that students may have in your clinical area. Try to think of as many as you can. You might like to separate these into categories, for example medicines management activities, assessment activities, communication activities, etc.

Hopefully, you will have identified a large number of learning opportunities for students. It is likely that there will be opportunities that are suitable for students at different stages of their programme, for example first year, second year and third year students. It would be worthwhile to indicate in your list the level of the student that opportunities are most applicable for. This will help you decide the different groups of students that can and should be encouraged to undertake their clinical experience in your area.

KEY POINT

If your area has a student welcome folder, consider putting a list of learning opportunities and learning experiences in the folder. Students will find this a valuable resource, and it will reassure them that they will be encouraged to learn as much as possible while on their placement.

THE NON-LEARNING ENVIRONMENT

It is not uncommon for mentors to facilitate students on placement without thinking through the learning opportunities that are available for them and how appropriate they all may be. If your placement area has been supporting students for a number of years then it is best practice to regularly reconsider whether any of the learning opportunities have changed. Given that healthcare is in a constant state of change, it is not unreasonable to assume that the learning opportunities available to students will also be likely to fluctuate.

By undertaking Activity 3.3 you should have identified the majority of learning opportunities that are available for students in your practice area. However, it may be that there are not as many learning opportunities as you assumed, or perhaps the opportunities are more suitable to a particular group of student. For example, the learning opportunities you have may be best suited to third year students; however, you may be currently supporting first year or second year students. If this is the case then you must discuss this with your manager and/or contact the university to discuss appropriate student allocation. It benefits no-one if students are inappropriately placed in your area where there are limited learning opportunities available or the learning opportunities are not applicable to the level of the student.

PERSONAL PREPARATION

Assuming that you work in a practice area that is suitable for students to achieve their learning outcomes, the next step is to ensure that you are personally prepared for your role and responsibility as a mentor. Once again, you cannot assume that this will all just fall into place once a student is allocated to you, and being personally prepared is your own responsibility – no one can or should be expected to do this for you.

AM I COMPETENT?

In the UK it is the NMC that sets the professional standard that is expected of a mentor. As part of this professional accountability you are required to undertake a self-assessment of your competence to be a mentor on a yearly basis. If you fall short of the standard expected of a mentor the NMC would expect you to take measures to rectify this prior to you undertaking a mentorship role. This has already been discussed extensively in Chapter 2. Take the time now to review these standards if you have not already done so (see Appendix).

Remember that maintaining an up-to-date record of your mentoring experiences and record of your attendances at mentor updates is all part of the evidence required by the NMC to demonstrate that you have adequately prepared for your role as a mentor. In essence, all these measures are there to ensure that mentors are competent to undertake their role of facilitating and assessing students on clinical placement. These standards therefore are an integral part of your pre-practice preparation for a student.

Remember too that the NMC would expect that you are a competent practitioner within your own clinical specialty prior to mentoring a student. You will not be in a position to facilitate learning or identify student competence if you yourself are not competent in your professional role. You should ensure therefore that prior to undertaking the mentorship of a student that you are up-to-date in your annual professional performance review.

DO I UNDERSTAND THE STUDENTS TRAINING PROGRAMME?

If you are expecting students in your area then part of your preparation is to ensure that you are up-to-date with the current programme requirements for the students you will be mentoring. At the very least you will need to have a general understanding of the taught content of the programme, the current educational level of the students you will be mentoring and the purpose of the practice placement they will be undertaking with you. Not only will this knowledge aid you in planning learning experiences during the placement, it will also assist you in determining expectations for competence. This information should be a part of your preparation before students arrive in your clinical area, not left until students have actually arrived.

If you are unsure of this information then there are various ways of finding it out. The university will have provided your practice area with information regarding their students' programme. This may be in the form of a website, booklet or perhaps even on a CD or memory stick. Universities provide this information in a number of different ways, and it is likely that it will also be covered during face-to-face mentor updates. It may be that you already have this information, but it has been relegated to a bookshelf where it is currently collecting dust. The fact that you might have this information does not mean that you are prepared for a student's arrival. It is your responsibility to access and read this information prior to students arriving in your placement so you are adequately prepared.

KEY POINT

Consider creating a mentor resource folder for your clinical area. It can be a fast way to access materials and information supplied by the university on the students programme.

DO I UNDERSTAND THE REQUIREMENTS FOR ENTRY TO THE REGISTER?

The NMC provides information regarding the pre-registration nursing programme and the standards of proficiency expected on completion of that programme. These documents are readily available on the NMC website at http://www.nmc-uk.org/.

If you have not already done so then take the time now to access and read any documents related to standards of competence set by the NMC. They will provide you with an overview of the requirements for the pre-registration programme for nurses and also the competency level that has been pre-determined by the NMC. In the next chapter we will look at the competency required by students in far more detail, however, for now, you should use the NMC standards as a guide in your preparation as a mentor for student placement.

We already know that your role as a mentor is twofold. First, you will be required to facilitate student learning while they are with you on their placement. Second, you will be required to assess their competence. You must therefore have a very good understanding of what it is that students are required to learn, and the expectations for competence as determined by the NMC before the student arrives for their practice placement. Without this information you will be unable to fulfil either of your mentoring roles, and waiting until the student arrives to seek out this information will waste valuable time; theirs and yours.

DO I UNDERSTAND MY ACCOUNTABILITY AND RESPONSIBILITY AS A MENTOR?

A vital part of your personal preparation for students is ensuring that you are familiar with and understand your professional accountability and responsibility as a mentor. The NMC has outlined this information within the *Standards to Support Learning and Assessment in Practice* (NMC, 2008). This can be accessed at http://www.nmc-uk.org/. In particular you should pay attention to the following:

- Section 3.2.4
- Section 3.2.5
- Section 3.2.6.

These sections outline the requirement for applying the NMC mentor standards in practice. If you have not already read this information then it is highly recommended that you do so. There is no substitute in reading for yourself the NMC's expectations for you in this role.

DO I KNOW HOW TO ACCESS SUPPORT?

Being a mentor can be a challenging experience and prior to a student arriving in your practice area you should make yourself aware of the support mechanisms available to you with regards to your role. The support available to you may come in a variety of forms.

Most universities supply mentors with a wide range of paper and electronic resources that can be used to support the mentoring role. Such resources may include the following:

- mentor information books
- information on cd-roms or memory sticks
- pocket guides
- mentor newsletters
- mentor guidance sheets and policies
- mentor websites provided by the university.

In addition, most universities provide mentors with a network of people that may be contacted by mentors for support during student placement. These may include:

- link lecturers
- programme leaders
- practice educators/facilitators/advisors.

Very often the lecturers will be involved in visits to the clinical area at scheduled times, or provide a drop-in clinic or surgery. In addition, your organization may also provide resources or people who can support you in your mentoring role. These may include:

- placement facilitators
- managers
- practice educators
- lecturer practitioners
- senior mentors.

It is your responsibility as a mentor to ensure that you are aware of all the support mechanisms available to you prior to students commencing clinical placement. You should be aware of what the specific resources available to you are, who to contact, and how to contact them before students arrive.

GENERAL PLANNING

Before students arrive in your practice area there needs to be some specific planning undertaken to ensure everyone is ready for their arrival. Remember our example of the best-case scenario? This ideal can only be reached if everyone works together and there are clear channels of communication.

HOW DO I KNOW WHEN TO EXPECT STUDENTS?

It is the responsibility of the university to allocate students to their practice placement. If students are allocated to your clinical area then a senior person within your organization, perhaps a ward or unit manager, would have agreed this with the university. Before a student's arrival in the clinical area the university is required to inform your placement of the following:

- when the student will be arriving
- the name of the student
- the length of placement
- the level of the student (first year, second year, etc.)
- any study days planned during the placement.

The information regarding a student's arrival will be passed on either through a letter, email or website. Each practice area will have been informed by the university how they can expect to receive this information and what they are required to do to access it. However, it is the responsibility of 'somebody' in practice to ensure that this information is accessed, and then shared amongst your staff so that everyone is aware of who to expect and when they are expected. If students arrive unexpectedly in your clinical area then there are three possible explanations for this.

The most common explanation is that while 'someone' should be aware of a student's arrival, the system has failed in some way and either 'nobody' has accessed this information or the information has not been passed on. In either case, best practice in this circumstance is for this information to be checked as soon as is possible by someone in the clinical area against the records supplied by the university. While this information is being checked it is very important that the student is welcomed and the disruption minimized. Remember that the student will be feeling very nervous anyway, and if they are made to feel unwanted this will only exacerbate their anxiety.

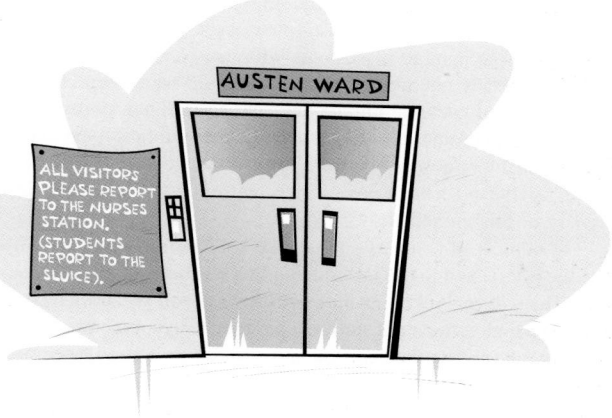

It may be that the university has inadvertently forgotten to pass on this information, or the information is sitting in an unread email. Once again, someone in the clinical area should check with the university to ascertain if the student is expected. It is for this reason that knowing who and how to contact the university is a vital part of preparing for students. In any case, while the information is being checked the student should be welcomed and made to feel at ease.

The last option is that the student has turned up to the wrong place. This is also quite common, especially if the student is new to your organization or has had limited experience of clinical placement. If it is found that they are in the wrong placement then you should make the effort to minimize this mistake and redirect them to where they should be with kindness. Anyone can make a mistake, and if a student is made to feel stupid they will quickly lose confidence. Try to laugh it off with them and offer help where possible to find out where they should be. Common courtesy goes a long way here; just remember how you would feel.

KEY POINT

A student notice board or resource folder is a great way to advertise when students are expected. If they are kept up to date mentors can be easily informed and students will feel welcome and wanted.

HOW MANY STUDENTS SHOULD I EXPECT?

Along with the information regarding when to expect students, would have been an agreement regarding capacity. The term *capacity* is used to identify the number of students who can be on practice placement in your area at any one time. The university will have been informed about the capacity of your ward/unit/ clinic, etc. to facilitate students. This number is used to ensure that students are distributed fairly and that there are enough mentors at any one time to facilitate student numbers on placement. If your placement capacity changes then you must inform the university of this immediately.

The number of students you receive and the frequency of students will be directly related to the information that has been supplied to the university. The university will not automatically know if you have recently experienced a high turnover of staff that has reduced your mentor numbers; you will have to update them on this information well in advance of students being allocated to your area. This must be a reasonable amount of time to allow the university to find the student an alternative practice placement.

PRE-PLACEMENT VISITS

The university is required to provide advanced notice of a student's placement in your practice area. The notice period should be at least 6 weeks but could even be many months depending on the university systems. Where this is the case it is best practice to encourage pre-placement visits for students. These are beneficial for both students and mentors, and can facilitate the following:

- introductions and building a rapport
- orientation to the layout of the practice area
- confirmation of shift times, shift patterns and travel arrangements.

A pre-placement visit should be viewed as an informal opportunity for a student and mentor to meet. Very often it can be arranged over the telephone, or in some cases via email. It does not have to be a lengthy period of time, around 15–30 minutes is usually more than adequate. If you can, try to provide your student with their off-duty for at least the first week of placement and confirm with them where they should report to on the first day of their placement. If there are any special considerations that the student may not be aware of, for example parking arrangements, then ensure your student is informed. Taking the time to meet a student prior to the placement will pay dividends in the long term; not only will they arrive on the placement feeling welcome, they will already feel that you care about them and their learning experience.

ALLOCATING A MENTOR

One of the key features of preparing for student placement involves allocating a mentor to each student in advance of the placement commencing. Not only is this best practice from a practical point of view, it is also recommended by the NMC. If mentors and students are allocated prior to the placement commencing, this allows for thorough preparation by both. It also ensures that some thought has been put into the capacity of the mentor to facilitate the student's learning and assessment for the full placement period. Ideally, the mentor should not have any extended leave during the placement, for example holidays or study leave as happens in Case study 3.2.

If the allocation of the mentor is not planned then this can end up being a rushed decision with little thought put into whether the mentor will be able to support the student. In these circumstances facilitation of learning and assessment can quickly descend into chaos, and under such circumstances poor decisions are often made.

Case study 3.2 *A mentor speaks of being allocated a student*

'I remember one placement where a student came up to me on her first day and said that the manager had decided I was the mentor. I thought at the time it was odd because I was off on a two-week holiday the next week. I should have said something, but I just thought the manager knew what she was doing. Anyway, it turns out she had just forgotten about my leave. I came back from holidays straight onto nights, and didn't see my student again. I'm not sure what happened to her, I guess someone else took over.'

PLANNING THE OFF-DUTY

The only way to guarantee that you are able to supervise your student adequately while they are on practice placement is to ensure that they are matched to your off-duty. In working identical shifts you will have the maximum opportunity of facilitating learning experiences and also give yourself a chance to undertake ongoing assessment of their competence. You will also be able to accurately record the number of hours they have attended placement, with sicknesses and absences tracked carefully. Both you and your student will benefit equally from this arrangement and it works especially well if the mentor is allocated prior to the placement beginning, as this also ensures that the mentor is able to greet the student on their first day of placement. The NMC requires that students make themselves available for the full range of 24/7 shifts so that they can experience all aspects of patient care. This requirement should make it a simple process to match a student's off-duty with that of their mentor for the entire placement period. This will have the added benefit of ensuring that the mentor will be available for the full placement experience, and that a booked holiday or period of study leave has not been forgotten.

It may be that it is not always possible for mentors and students to work every shift together. When this is the case, it is best practice for a student to be allocated a co-mentor, someone who can supervise the student and feedback progress to the named mentor as required. A word of caution here, however; it is poor practice to allow students to select or nominate their own off-duty, as this can lead to minimal supervision during the placement (see Case study 3.3). You must remember that students are required to attend practice placements so a mentor can facilitate their learning and assess their competence. They are not simply on the placement to complete a set number of hours. Students who make special

Case study 3.3 *Mentors and students working together*

Caroline is an experienced mentor, she enjoys facilitating student learning and always ensures that her student is allocated the same off-duty so they can maximize their time working together. On the first day of placement Caroline and her student Eunice discuss the off-duty for the first two weeks of the placement. Caroline and Eunice will be working a mix of weekday and weekend long day (LD) shifts together. She has planned the first two weeks to ensure that they will spend approximately 75 hours working together and there will be plenty of opportunities to conduct the initial interview and give feedback.

Their off-duty is planned as follows:

Week 1

	Mon	Tues	Wed	Thur	Fri	Sat	Sun
Caroline	LD		LD			LD	LD
Eunice	LD		LD			LD	LD

Week 2

	Mon	Tues	Wed	Thur	Fri	Sat	Sun
Caroline		LD	LD		LD		
Eunice		LD	LD		LD		

Eunice is very unhappy when she is given this off-duty. She explains to Caroline that she has no-one to care for her children on a weekend and so she must always have these days off. She also states that she cannot work on a Friday, but can do Thursday nights (N) instead. Although unhappy with this arrangement Caroline does not want to appear uncaring so she allows Eunice to alter the off-duty to the following.

Week 1

	Mon	Tues	Wed	Thur	Fri	Sat	Sun
Caroline	LD		LD			LD	LD
Eunice	LD		LD	LD			

Week 2

	Mon	Tues	Wed	Thur	Fri	Sat	Sun
Caroline		LD	LD		LD		
Eunice	LD	LD		N			

Continued

- a profile of the staff working in the area – a 'who's who', including the multidisciplinary team
- contact details of relevant people – for example link lecturers
- a brief description of the type of placement/specialty
- learning opportunities for students (you may wish to split these into opportunities for first, second and third years)
- some recommended further reading that is related to the specialty.

Unless there is some specific reason for doing so, try not to include policies in a student folder. While there is no doubt that policies are important, they are not exactly the most stimulating documents to read. It would be hard for a student to see how a 50-page policy on health and safety within a student folder is your way of welcoming them to the practice placement. They will feel far more welcome if you tell them you care about their health and safety and provide them access to these policies within the workplace. It is far better to list within the folder where policies may be accessed if required. Many organizations now provide policies via intranet sites. If this is the case then the student folder should contain details of how they may access these policies, including usernames and passwords if required.

STUDENT NOTICEBOARDS

Many practice areas allocate a specific section or separate noticeboard for student information. This is a great idea and can be very useful for students if it contains good, relevant and up-to-date information that is actually of help. However, because a noticeboard is very visual it can very quickly become a negative rather than a positive. If a student walks into your unit on the first day and is greeted with an empty student noticeboard or information that is three years old it may imply they are unwelcome and not cared about. If you are going to have a noticeboard then this must be kept very current and updated on a regular basis. In fact it is better not to have a noticeboard for students at all, than have one that is badly utilized. If you are going to have a student noticeboard then you could consider providing the following information:

- link lecturer details and availability
- details of student drop-in clinics or student surgeries available locally
- upcoming talks, lectures, teaching sessions within your organization that students may be able to attend
- names of students, their mentors and dates when initial, mid and final interviews are due.

Remember that a student noticeboard does not have to be huge; it is far better to have a small amount of relevant information than vast quantities of pointless notices.

KEY POINT

If you have never had a student noticeboard before, start very small and build up slowly. Try starting with an area no bigger than A1 and make sure that someone is prepared to review the noticeboard regularly to ensure that the information is current, useful and interesting.

UPDATING STUDENT INFORMATION

No matter what resource is being used in your area to provide information for students, it will have little value if it is not kept up-to-date. Someone specific in your clinical area will need to be designated with the responsibility of maintaining and updating the information for any resource you have. Maintaining student resources must also happen as part of the preparation for students, so it will need to be constantly monitored.

Ideally this should be a voluntary role, someone who already has a keen interest in students and wants to promote your unit in the best possible context to students. Your unit will need to think very carefully about what resources to provide, and then commit to keeping these up-to-date. For example, if keeping the information on a student noticeboard current is proving far too time consuming, then take this down and concentrate on maintaining a good resource folder.

GETTING STUDENT PREPARATION RIGHT

No matter how much preparation you may have done for a student's placement there will always be occasions when somehow the system falls down. This is rarely a deliberate act; however, this fact does not make a student feel better when they arrive and are clearly not expected. If you have not already done so it may be useful to develop a checklist or guide of areas that need to be regularly monitored to ensure that your area is prepared for students. Making this a part of your staff management routine can ensure that facilitating students runs as smoothly as possible. Box 3.1 provides a sample of a student preparation checklist.

Box 3.1 Preparing for students checklist

	Yes/No
Are there enough mentors for the number of students we have agreed to support?	☐
Are sufficient mentors up-to-date to support the student numbers agreed?	☐
Is there a process for finding out when students are arriving?	☐
Are pre-placement visits encouraged?	☐
Is a named mentor allocated prior to the student starting the placement?	☐
Are the mentor and student rostered to work together?	☐
Are the mentor and student rostered together on the first day?	☐
Is there a named contact at the university if there are any issues that arise?	☐
Is there a process in place to ensure our student resources are kept up-to-date?	☐

While there is no guarantee that a checklist will prevent all problems, it will assist in troubleshooting the most common areas where student preparation may be overlooked. Get this right and the placement can start under the best possible circumstances.

PREPARATION IS THE KEY

In this chapter we have discussed many aspects of preparing for students in a practice area. We have looked at personal preparation and also preparation from the perspective of a practice area. While we have dedicated a whole chapter to the issue of preparing for students, the fact is that most of the issues addressed are not time consuming or costly. On the whole, many of the issues addressed are a simple matter of common sense. However, it would be safe to say that for most mentors preparing for students is the one area of their role that they consistently overlook or put the least effort into addressing. Ironically, inadequate preparation is the main reason why a student's practice placement may be less than satisfactory. The plain fact is that preparation for placement does matter, and should be considered as the key to success.

TOP TIPS

- Develop a strategy for student preparation; prepare yourself and your practice area.
- Keep yourself up-to-date and competent as a mentor; address outstanding areas of knowledge before mentoring students.
- Consider how to welcome students; either by developing welcome packs or noticeboards and arranging pre-placement visits.
- Develop a 'Student preparation checklist' and ensure it is implemented at regular intervals.

CHAPTER 4

UNDERSTANDING THE PRACTICE ASSESSMENT DOCUMENT

Chapter Aims

The purpose of this chapter is to explore the practice assessment document and the meaning of learning outcomes in more depth. After reading this chapter you will be able to:

- Explain the role of the practice assessment document in the student's learning experience.
- Identify the key documents which state the level of competence a student must meet in order to enter the branch programme and the register.
- Problem solve the meaning of learning outcomes and plan learning accordingly.

THE PRACTICE ASSESSMENT DOCUMENT

Every student will come to their placement with a practice assessment document of some description. This document may be referred to as any of the following:

- clinical skills book
- assessment book
- assessment of practice record
- practice learning document
- placement assessment document.

Effectively, these documents or booklets are all the same thing because they have the same purpose as a record of the student's learning and the mentor's assessment. The structure and content will vary differently depending on the university; however, there are core features and it is one of these, the learning outcomes, which will be explored in this chapter. To ensure clarity and understanding the document will be referred to as the practice assessment document or PAD within this chapter.

Box 4.1 Key features of practice assessment documents

Core features
- Student and placement details page
- Instructions on how to complete the booklet
- A list of learning outcomes
- Space to record assessment interviews
- Space to record the outcome of the assessment
- Ongoing Achievement Record.

Optional extras
- Space for a second attempt at practice to be documented
- Timesheet
- Contact details of university placements department or link lecturer
- Clinical skills advice detailing what the student can or can't do
- Incident/accident form
- List of skills to be obtained
- Space to record action plans
- Space to record testimonies from other healthcare professionals, service users, etc.

A PAD is a record of what the university requires the student to achieve in practice in order to meet the standards the NMC requires for entry to the branch and the register. The PAD will become a record of the learning the student has undertaken and the mentor's assessment of that learning.

Within the PAD there will be a list of learning outcomes, competencies or proficiencies, which are required to be assessed by the mentor and achieved by the student to progress further in their training. There could be statements or grids to be filled in requiring the mentor's signatures and dates for verification of learning undertaken by the student. Box 4.1 represents some of the key features included within most PADs.

LAYOUT OF THE PRACTICE ASSESSMENT DOCUMENT

PADs are developed by universities and provided to students before they attend placement. Although the content of a PAD is usually quite similar across universities, the layout and structure will be very different. There is no universal template for PADs, and as a result, universities are responsible for developing their own documents according to their interpretation of NMC guidelines.

All PADs will be structured to allow mentors to follow the practice assessment process. As a result they will all contain sections for documentation of interviews with students (initial, midpoint, final). However, there will be variable amounts of space allocated within the document where mentors are required to document progress.

In addition, many PADs allocate sections where students are required to maintain records, perhaps as reflective journals, evidence of achieving competence or commentaries related to their practice placement experience. In both cases the PAD should clearly indicate where mentors and students are to maintain records and what types of records should be maintained.

The PAD will also contain instructions detailing the mentor's role in completing the book. It is essential to read or re-read these instructions as lack of familiarity with the book, and what is required of the mentor, can lead to errors. Errors made by mentors in the PAD can result in questions being asked about the accuracy of the assessment process, causing the student additional anxiety (see Case study 4.1).

DOCUMENTING ASSESSMENT

Obviously the PAD will contain a section where a mentor is required to carry out an assessment. Usually this will mean signing or initialling your name against a list of competencies. You may be required to decide if learning outcomes have been achieved or not achieved; in some cases you may even be expected to grade a student according to a marking grid or pre-determined criteria set by the university. Regular mentor updating should ensure that you are familiar with the system used by your university in assessing students, so this is a vital aspect of your preparation before the student arrives. The PAD should also contain instructions regarding the assessment process required, so you should take the time to read this and clarify any areas you are unsure about.

Case study 4.1 A mentor speaks of her experience in documenting within a PAD

'When I first became a mentor I didn't really understand the importance of documenting within the student's assessment book. I remember that students would show me their books and I would sign my name against their

Continued

Case study 4.1 A mentor speaks of her experience in documenting within a PAD—Cont'd

learning objectives without hesitation. For some reason I thought that I was signing to say that I agreed to assess the student on all the things listed in the book and never gave it a second thought. Then one day I overheard two students talking in the corridor and they were basically laughing and saying that it was easy to pass with me, I'd sign their books without even assessing them. I literally broke out in a sweat. For months I'd been signing students as competent without even realizing it. I just felt so stupid. As soon as I looked in the book I realized that the instructions were there, I had just never bothered to read them. I'd not gone to my mentor update either; it just wasn't one of my priorities. Safe to say I learnt my lesson the hard way. I make a point now of reading everything about the assessment just to make sure I'm getting it right. As far as I'm concerned it's worth the extra ten minutes to have peace of mind that I'm getting it right.'

LEARNING CONTRACTS

Most PADs will contain an area for mentors and students to develop learning contracts. Learning contracts are an agreement between the mentor and the student detailing what both parties are to do to enable the student to learn. They are sometimes referred to as action plans or development plans. As we will discover in Chapter 5, the initial interview is an ideal time to develop a learning contract. There may be other occasions such as the midpoint interview when learning contracts are useful. Likewise, learning contracts are vital if a student is underperforming or a new learning opportunity has arisen and it is necessary to document an agreement as to how the student will engage with this learning. There will usually be space in the PAD to document the learning contracts. Sometimes these are included as pre-printed templates within the PAD, often coinciding with the formal interview stages.

WHAT IF I RUN OUT OF SPACE TO DOCUMENT?

When designing a PAD, universities will try to predict the amount of space required by mentors to complete the required assessment documentation. If the space required is not sufficient then it is advisable to contact a link lecturer from the university who will discuss the options open to you. As the PAD is a formal assessment document it is important that all relevant information is recorded, and not simply left out due to a lack of writing space. It may be that you are advised to record additional documentation on headed paper, giving a copy to the student and the link lecturer if necessary.

KEY POINT

Documented learning contracts provide evidence towards the assessment process being followed and are useful for those occasions where the student is not performing to the required level and will provide evidence of the difficulties the student has encountered.

You may find that more space is required within a PAD if a mentor or student identifies a specific learning need which could impact on the student's ability to achieve one or more learning outcomes. If there are multiple issues being addressed then the learning contract or action plan may be quite lengthy in order to specifically address that need.

For example, a student could be struggling with their documentation skills, as reflected in their nursing notes, assessments, care plans, discharges and/or referrals. To enable the student to develop these skills alongside the other learning opportunities you could document an action plan that included some of the following aspects:

- using an English and nursing dictionary when writing records
- using the 16 Principles of Good Record Keeping listed in the NMC's guidance on Record Keeping as a checklist for their documentation
- writing rough copies of documentation so that you can check the work and provide feedback
- using your organization's policy on record keeping to critique other professionals' entries.

If your plan for supporting the student is quite detailed with a number of aspects and variables then the resulting learning contract may also require considerable space in order to document it fully. Don't be afraid to document what is required as there is no standard for how much documentation each student will require to support their learning.

USING THE PRACTICE ASSESSMENT DOCUMENT DURING PLACEMENT

Students can be very protective regarding their PADs, as replacing the document can be quite difficult if lost. For this reason students may avoid regularly bringing their PAD to placement for fear of losing or damaging it. They may bring in photocopies of what they perceive as the relevant pages. It is not uncommon for students to have one PAD that will cover several placements, modules or years in the programme and the corresponding practice assessments for these placements. The student's response to protect the PAD is understandable when the state of the PAD is viewed as a reflection of the student's presentation and organizational skills.

While anxiety about their PAD is understandable it is not acceptable for a student to ask you to fill in the photocopied sheets or decline for you to see and write in the original. To avoid anxiety it is a good idea to establish with the student at the beginning of the placement what access you will require to their PAD and where it may be safely stored to prevent damage (see Case study 4.2).

Case study 4.2 A mentor's experience of using the PAD

'On the first day of the placement I discussed with my student that I would need to have access to his PAD regularly throughout the placement so we could review his learning outcomes together. This seemed to really worry him and he stated that he would prefer not to bring his PAD to placement. He explained that his mentor the year before had taken his book home and it had been lost. He had a very difficult time getting a replacement copy and his learning during the placement had suffered as a result. Once I knew what the problem was the solution was easy. I showed him a locker on the ward where he could keep his book during the placement and supplied him with the combination lock. I assured him that we would always document in it together and that I would never want to take it away from him. Not only did we find a solution that suited us both, we were able to establish a level of trust and respect from the very beginning.'

WRITING IN THE PAD

When writing in the PAD it is essential to view the document as important as any other nursing record. The NMC's guidance for record keeping should be followed. Keep statements clear and factual; avoid unspecific generic sentences which could lead to misunderstandings and sign and date in every space required. Be specific about any agreements with the student; for example state exactly what the student must do for each learning outcome rather than 'we have discussed and agreed what needs to be done to achieve the learning outcomes'. Remember what you write could be available for the next mentor but also for the student for the rest of their programme, and therefore needs to be constructive and useful.

As stated earlier, the PAD records two essential elements related to the student's placement; the outcome of the assessment and the processes taken to ensure the assessment is valid and reliable. Even if process has been followed, a failure to record accurately in the PAD can make it very difficult to prove at a later date if correct assessment processes have been followed. Therefore what you write needs to withstand outside scrutiny.

LEARNING OUTCOMES

Every summative assessment of a student's learning in practice will have a list of learning outcomes which the mentor will be required to assess. Learning outcomes are statements which identify what the student must learn, know and be able to perform. The outcomes will focus on the knowledge, skills and professional attitude required of the student at that level. The final assessment interview in the placement requires mentors to make the final decision as to the achievement of the learning outcomes to the standard required.

The learning outcomes will be mapped against the proficiencies required by the NMC. They are responsible for setting the standard for pre-registration nursing programmes in the UK. In some cases the learning outcomes in the PAD will be taken directly from standards within their documents, in others they could be a statement encompassing more than one of the standards or competencies listed. Now undertake Activity 4.1.

Activity 4.1 Learning outcomes

Access the NMC website at www.nmc-uk.org and review the current standards related to pre-registration nursing. Now have a look at some of the learning outcomes that are in the PADs you are assessing. Make a list of at least three different outcomes. Can you identify if the learning outcomes you are required to assess in your placement are taken directly from one of the identified documents or are an amalgamation of the competencies listed?

Outcome 1

Outcome 2

Outcome 3

Some learning outcomes will be very specific, with a clear expectation of what is to be achieved in a specific placement or in every placement. For example, a learning outcome might state something like:

The student must safely and competently administer five intramuscular injections.

In this example the learning outcome is very clear because the roles of the student and the mentor are very well defined. The learning outcome requires you to verify that the student is competent in a certain skill. Most mentors would feel quite confident with this type of learning outcome as it gives explicit direction on what is required.

Other learning outcomes however may be broad and open for interpretation. These types of learning outcomes provide a student with the freedom to achieve these in any clinical area. A broad learning outcome has the advantage of not restricting the types of opportunities that must be available for the student. Broad outcomes help to maximize the possibility of the student achieving the standard required.

However, these learning outcomes often pose difficulties for mentors as the interpretation of exactly what is required to be learnt and then what evidence the student must produce to demonstrate competence may not be immediately apparent. It would be fair to say that the broader the learning outcome the more difficult it is for a mentor to interpret. Conversely, the broader the outcome the easier it becomes for the student to achieve.

KEY POINT

There will usually be similarities in the types of learning outcomes students attempt in your practice area. If any outcomes are routinely used that require interpretation discuss these with other mentors in your area to ensure that your expectations and interpretations have a similar focus.

As part of the initial interview the mentor must discuss with their student how the learning outcomes can be achieved in the placement. This will involve identifying the learning opportunities available for the student and what evidence is required to demonstrate competence and achievement of the learning outcomes. Quite simply your expectations of a student must be mapped against a learning outcome. If your expectations of a student cannot be mapped against an outcome then you are basing your assessment on your personal agenda.

The first step in this process is to understand what the learning outcome actually means; this may involve interpreting some of the language related to the assessment and, if necessary, splitting the outcome into smaller sections so that it becomes more meaningful and measureable. After understanding what the learning outcome requires you to assess, the mentor must also identify learning opportunities and the evidence required to demonstrate competence. The latter two stages are far easier if you have been able to grasp what the learning outcome requires you to do.

The SMART acronym outlined in Box 4.2 may be familiar to you. It is a principle applied to care plans on a daily basis and one that should also be applied to learning outcomes. If you do encounter a learning outcome which is difficult to interpret, then applying the SMART principles will be invaluable. By applying these principles you will be able to split the outcome into more understandable sections which will also ensure you can clarify with the student what it is you want them to learn. Your understanding of learning outcomes will naturally improve as you become more familiar with the terminology used.

Box 4.2 The SMART acronym

Specific	States what the student is expected to achieve in terms of knowledge and skills, which might be intellectual or practical skills, and attitudes and values.
Measurable	Observable and assessable, i.e. clearly state the behaviour the student will demonstrate to show they have achieved the outcome.
Achievable	Within the student's range of abilities.
Relevant	Appropriate to the knowledge and skill level expected of the student.
Time scaled	Clear target dates set for achievement.

TRANSLATING THE JARGON

Interpreting what a learning outcome means can be challenging because not all the proficiencies and competencies are written using terminology in everyday language. Yet, mentors are required to be familiar enough with it to enable a student to access the relevant learning opportunities and then assess their learning against the learning outcomes.

When translating what the outcome means to you, it makes sense to start with the words which frequently appear as verbs within learning outcomes. The translation must also relate to a clinical learning experience rather than a straight and direct definition from a dictionary. There are some examples provided in Box 4.3. Now undertake Activity 4.2.

Activity 4.2 Understanding learning outcomes

In Activity 4.1 you made a list of three learning outcomes that you are required to assess in your clinical area. Are there any verbs that appear frequently in the learning outcomes you are required to assess? What is your understanding of these verbs?

KEY POINT

It is useful to keep a list and definitions of commonly used verbs within PADs in your practice area. This will help to ensure all mentors in the practice placement are assessing students according to the same criteria.

IDENTIFICATION OF LEARNING OPPORTUNITIES

A significant part of a mentor's role is to facilitate student access to learning opportunities. In Chapter 5 we will discuss the different ways that mentors can do this. Therefore it is essential that mentors and students understand exactly what a learning outcome requires them to do, as this will be the foundation for planning future learning experiences. We have already discussed that some learning outcomes will clearly indicate what learning opportunities the student could access. Some are less clear; and will require further interpretation before progress can be made. Boxes 4.4 and 4.5 illustrate the differences between the two different types of learning outcomes.

Box 4.3 Verbs and their meaning in the clinical learning context

The following list provides some examples of common verbs used within learning outcomes. It is not exhaustive but a good place to start as it not only gives an idea of how students could make the most of the learning opportunity but also hints towards what sort of evidence you could ask of the student.

Verb	Meaning and interpretation
Describe	Requires the student to prove what knowledge they have for example relating to a specific assessment, intervention, diagnosis, medication.
Demonstrate	Requires the student to be able to perform a skill or apply knowledge and understanding of concepts and theories related to clinical practice.
Recognizes	Requires the student to differentiate between what was expected and what was not expected but may not have the language to define the differences or the skills to respond.
Acts	Requires the student to perform in a given manner that is professionally expected.
Supports	Requires the student to help, assist and make suggestions.
Identify	Requires a student to see and be able to name the differences.
Manage	Requires a student to perform a given task accurately, safely, and professionally.
Applies	Requires a student to choose or select the right intervention based upon a sound knowledge base and then be able to put this into practice.
Ensures	Requires a student to make sure that a given task is completed or that others do it.
Challenges	Requires a student to question, debate and provide evidence for discussion.
Establish	Requires a student to start, create or begin to develop such things as therapeutic relationships.
Maintain	Requires a student to perform to a given standard at all times once mastered the task, e.g. written documentation.
Participate	Requires a student to actively take part in a given aspect of patient care with others.
Contribute	Requires a student to make suggestions or add to discussions that facilitate care or the management of the clinical environment.

Box 4.4 A clear learning outcome

Learning Outcome: Demonstrates the ability to accurately perform drug calculations for intravenous medicine administration.

In other words, the student will need to perform drug calculations and apply knowledge and understanding of drug calculation formulas. Most mentors and students would understand this requirement from reading the learning outcome.

Box 4.5 A learning outcome requiring interpretation

Learning Outcome: Actively involves the patient/client in their assessment and care planning.

This learning outcome is a little more difficult to interpret. The verb 'actively' requires the student to take part, however there are no specific lists of assessment or care planning events that may be relevant. The learning outcome is deliberately non-specific to allow the mentor and student to discuss and agree appropriate assessment and care planning situations.

EVIDENCE

Evidence is what the student should produce to demonstrate competence; in other words proof that learning has taken place. This evidence should be directly related to the learning outcome and learning opportunities and the student must know what is expected of them right from the beginning. In Chapter 5 we will discuss the documentation required at the initial interview and how this relates to evidence of competence.

For the time being it is more important to understand that if you have been able to understand and communicate the meaning of the learning outcome effectively the evidence should neatly follow. The evidence the student produces should be tangible and directly observed during their placement. Depending on the outcome you may prefer that the evidence be quantifiable; for example accurate documentation of a specific number of care plans or nursing notes (see Case studies 4.3 and 4.4).

Case study 4.3 *A link lecturer's experience of planning learning outcomes*

'I had been invited by the mentor to meet with them and their current student over concerns about the student's performance. When I met with the student and mentor, I read the practice document. One of the learning outcomes was looking at the values, beliefs, compassion and understanding of the student towards patients, carers, family and friends. The mentor wanted the student to competently give two injections to two different clients as evidence for this learning outcome. It was a very difficult situation because the student felt the mentor was being very unfair and the mentor felt the student was not performing at the level required. From my point of view I felt that the main issue was that the mentor and student did not understand the learning outcome and as a result the student was struggling to achieve what was required. When I went through the outcome with them they both acknowledged that their individual expectations had been compromised as a direct result of not understanding what to do. We spent 5 minutes discussing the opportunities available to meet the outcome and both the mentor and student left the meeting confident that competence could be easily demonstrated and achieved.'

PULLING IT ALTOGETHER

Once a verb is understood it becomes easier to identify what the learning outcome means in practice. There are several steps that are required in order to ensure you understand each learning outcome. These include:

Step 1 – Identify and understand the relevant verb used in the learning outcome.

Step 2 – Decide if the outcome needs breaking down so that it is manageable – use the SMART principles to rewrite the learning outcome so that you can understand it.

Step 3 – Look for any hints of types of learning opportunities and identify the learning opportunities the student should engage with.

Step 4 – Decide on what evidence will demonstrate proof of learning.

In Boxes 4.6, 4.7 and 4.8 there are three examples of using a step-by-step approach to understanding learning outcomes.

If you do need to break down a learning outcome in order to understand it then remember that this is an opportunity to make the smaller

Box 4.6 Understanding learning outcomes: Example 1

Student Learning Outcome: Identifies factors that influence and maintain patient/client dignity.

Step 1 – Identify and understand the relevant verb used in the learning outcome.

The relevant verb here is *identifies*. This tells you that the student should be able to name and differentiate between the different factors which influence and maintain patient client dignity.

Step 2 – Decide if the outcome needs breaking down so that it is manageable.

In this case it doesn't need to be broken down due to the clarity of the outcome.

Step 3 – Look for any hints of types of learning opportunities and identify the learning opportunities the student should engage with.

Patient/client dignity hints at learning opportunities which involve care giving such as supporting a patient in bed to have a wash or writing care plans with patients which clearly state the patient preferences or wishes and reading the NMC and Department of Health publications on dignity.

Step 4 – Decide what evidence will demonstrate proof of learning.

The student could list the factors which influence and maintain privacy and dignity for four patients and a documented care plan for each patient clearly demonstrating their preferences, choices and decisions about their care.

Case study 4.4 A student speaks of a difficult placement experience

'My most difficult placement experience was related to my mentor just not understanding my learning outcomes. I had all these outcomes to achieve and she just kept saying things like –'I don't know what that means' or 'We don't do any of that here'. I remember there was one learning outcome where I needed to demonstrate that I could prepare a patient for an invasive procedure. She just kept saying 'You'll have to do that on a surgical ward' and it was so frustrating because every day on this ward patients were having endoscopies. She just had it in her head that an invasive procedure meant surgery and that was it. So I spent weeks preparing patients for endoscopies, you know, checklists, consent, fasting, scans, making sure they had the correct ID and she refused this as evidence of my competence. So frustrating.'

Box 4.7 Understanding learning outcomes: Example 2

Student Learning Outcome: Documents concerns and information about patients/clients that may be significant.

Step 1 – Identify and understand the relevant verb used in the learning outcome.

The relevant verb here is *documents*. This tells you that you will be required to assess the student on what they write.

Step 2 – Decide if the outcome needs breaking down so that it is manageable.

In this case it doesn't need to be broken down due to the clarity of the outcome.

Step 3 – Look for any hints of types of learning opportunities and identify the learning opportunities the student should engage with.

In this example opportunities will arise in care delivery, assessment of patient's health status, interactions with family, carers or other professionals, it could be a referral to another professional including bleeping a doctor and recording this in the notes.

Step 4 – Decide what evidence will demonstrate proof of learning.

This would be examples of documented evidence which is written to the standard set by the NMC for record keeping including nursing notes, care plans, referral forms.

---

learning outcomes more specific to the opportunities your clinical learning environment offers. The important thing to remember is that if you have broken the learning outcome into smaller elements the student must demonstrate competence for each smaller element for them to be competent at the overall set learning outcome.

Examples of evidence to demonstrate that the student has learnt from the experiences could be:

- feeding back to the team at handover or a ward round what has taken place, what they specifically did and the outcome
- making a referral to a medication education group or making an appointment with a doctor or pharmacist if the patient or carer requested further support from the multidisciplinary team
- documented evidence in the evaluation of a care plan or in the nursing notes.

Box 4.8 Understanding learning outcomes: Example 3

Student Learning Outcome: Under supervision involves patient/client and carers in administration self-administration of medicines.

Step 1 – Identify and understand the relevant verb used in the learning outcome.

The relevant verb here is *involves*. This means the student should do this jointly with the patient and/or carer and not impose their own assumptions, beliefs and opinions onto the patient or carer. They will also need to undertake this activity under the supervision of a nurse and cannot do this independently.

Step 2 – Decide if the outcome needs breaking down so that it is manageable.

In this case the learning outcome would benefit from being broken down due to the needs of patients and carers differing as well as the differences in administration by oneself and by another. Some possible smaller learning outcomes may include:

- under supervision involve a patient and carer in learning how to self administer and store insulin safely
- under supervision involve a patient in learning how to use a dosette box for self administration
- under supervision involve a carer in learning how to administer adrenaline in an emergency.

Step 3 – Look for any hints of types of learning opportunities and identify the learning opportunities the student should engage with.

In this example the learning opportunities would be those which involve the administration of medication, opportunities to educate patients and carers and/or teach administration techniques.

Step 4 – Decide what evidence will demonstrate proof of learning.

First, *under supervision* means that you have to witness or another nurse must witness the student engage in the learning opportunity, therefore the evidence must be verifiable.

KEY POINT

Working with colleagues to agree what the learning outcome means, the learning opportunities available and the evidence for each in advance of students coming to placement will increase the validity and reliability in the assessment as all the mentors work towards the same goals.

ASSESSING IN PRACTICE

No matter how committed you are to your mentoring role or the development of students, you will not meet the standard expected of you as a mentor if you do not understand a student's PAD. If used correctly, the PAD will guide you and your student through the placement, highlighting where attention is required to the key stages within the assessment process. The PAD will provide a context for the goals of the placement, the opportunities to be explored and signpost when and where achievements have been made. At the core of every successful practice assessment is a mentor who can understand and use a PAD competently.

TOP TIPS

- Take the time to read for yourself the key elements of the PAD you are using in your practice area. Don't rely on the interpretation of others who may be mistaken themselves.
- Talk to your link lecturer and ask them to clarify aspects of the PAD that you may be unfamiliar with.
- Attend mentor updates and discuss with other mentors your experiences of documenting within the PAD; share good practice.
- Make a list of commonly used learning outcomes that are commonly assessed in your area and ensure all mentors are following the same interpretation.

Further Reading

Department of Health (2006) *Best practice competencies and capabilities for pre-registration mental health nurses in England*. Central Office of Information, London.

Nursing and Midwifery Council (2010) *Standards for Pre-Registration Nursing Education*. NMC, London.

Nursing and Midwifery Council (2007) *Essential Skills Clusters (ESCs) for Pre-registration Nursing Programmes*, Annexe 2 to NMC Circular 07/2007. NMC, London.

CHAPTER 5

ORIENTATION AND THE INITIAL INTERVIEW

Chapter Aims

The purpose of this chapter is to gain an understanding of the process and purpose of the initial interview. After reading this chapter you will be able to:

- Identify the main features, purpose and processes that should be considered when conducting an initial interview.
- Understand the importance of planning learning experiences that cater for a wide variety of student learning styles.
- Plan effectively for the initial interview event.

MEETING YOUR STUDENT

In Chapter 3 we explored the preparation that should take place before a student arrives in your clinical area. The purpose of thorough preparation is to identify potential problems and ensure that the practice placement gets off to the best possible start for both you and your student. If you are properly prepared for your student's arrival then the initial meeting should be a relaxed and friendly event. Ideally, you may have had contact with the student previously, either though a pre-placement visit or via the phone or email.

The first meeting is your opportunity to welcome them to the placement area and ensure they feel wanted and welcome. You only have one chance to get this right, so it is really important that this is handled well as this first meeting will set the tone for the rest of the placement. No matter how much information they may have about the placement, they will still be feeling very nervous about this first encounter, and will remember every detail about it. This is your chance to shine.

ORIENTATION

One of the best ways to ensure that a student feels welcome to the practice placement is to orientate them to the placement environment as soon as possible. Ideally, orientation should be a staged process during the first day to ensure that the student is provided with all the information they require and that they are given the opportunity to ask questions that may be relevant to them.

Try to start the orientation by showing your student the essentials; where to put their bag/coat etc, and the location of staff lockers or changing rooms if relevant. If possible, arrange for this to take place within the first few minutes of them arriving in the placement. If you have got a student locker or locked cupboard available for valuables then make sure the student knows how to access this. Knowing where to put your personal property and how to access these items throughout the day will put them at ease very early on as it shows that you are interested in their welfare.

The next step in the orientation involves introducing your student to the other staff on shift that day. Let everyone know the student's name and the year of the programme they are on. It's a good idea to identify yourself to your colleagues as the student's mentor, and let everyone know how long the placement is. If you can do this during handover then this is the best option as you don't have to repeat the information throughout the day.

An introduction does not have to be long or complex, something simple will do such as:

'Hi everyone, I'd like to introduce you to Jenny. She's a third-year student and she is on placement with us for 6 weeks. Today's her first day and just to let everyone know I'm her mentor during the placement.'

A simple and friendly introduction will allow greetings to be swapped. You can encourage your colleagues to introduce themselves and what their role is, or you can go around the group and do this yourself. If your practice area routinely does a handover, encourage your student to join in and ensure your student is provided with the same materials as other staff.

The second part of orientation will be to ensure that the student is orientated to the work area and that health and safety issues are addressed. Try to make this as informal as possible, without forgetting essential information. The types of information your student will need are:
- location of toilets/changing facilities
- location of fire exits and emergency equipment/evacuation procedures
- location of tea rooms, canteens, vending machines, etc.
- location of storerooms, treatment rooms, training rooms, etc.

Lastly, it is important that the student is aware of how to contact the placement, who to contact, and their off-duty for the placement. All these areas can be addressed throughout the first day to ensure that the student receives a thorough orientation without feeling overwhelmed.

KEY POINT

If your placement area has a student folder try to include some of the orientation information in here. Phone numbers and key staff in the placement are very useful to include. On the first day you can ask them to read the information in the folder and then ask any questions they may have.

INITIAL INTERVIEW

The initial interview is the first opportunity that you and your student will have to plan and discuss what is expected on the placement. Not only is it a chance to discuss each other's expectations, it also marks the beginning of the student's assessment. For this reason it is highly recommended that you do not try to schedule the initial interview for the first day of placement as your student will be taking in so much new information they will be unlikely to benefit (see Case study 5.1).

Case study 5.1 A student speaks about her first day of placement

'I started placement with a community psychiatric nurse and within the first hour she was pushing me to sit down for the initial interview. I just felt so overwhelmed and disorientated. She treated the interview like a task she had to get out of the way. As soon as we started the interview I knew the placement was going to be a disaster. She told me a little bit about the clinic where we would be based and asked me what I wanted to learn and that was about it. The whole interview lasted less than 10 minutes. I wanted to talk about my learning outcomes and show her my assessment book but it was obvious she was in a real rush and I felt too nervous to stand up for myself. That was my worst placement experience. Over half the placement went by before my mentor actually realized what it was I should have been learning and bothered to look at my assessment book. By the time she understood what I was meant to be learning I had missed a lot of learning opportunities and as a result I got very little useful feedback. What a waste.'

PLANNING THE INITIAL INTERVIEW

It is best practice to stage the initial interview in the first week of placement. If possible try to decide the date and time of the initial interview during the student's first day of placement so that you can both plan for the event. If you are both working the same off-duty then scheduling the initial interview during a shift that you are both working together in the first week should not be difficult.

When scheduling the initial interview try to allow at least one hour of protected time. This is not to say that the interview will always take one hour; however, by identifying this time you are creating a fixed period of time that can be planned for within the workload of others. You may want to consider planning the initial interview for a day in the first week when you know there is a senior staff skill mix, or a day that is typically quieter than others (Case study 5.2).

Case study 5.2 Scheduling an initial interview

Jones ward is a very busy surgical unit. In the past it was common practice for students to miss out on their initial interviews with mentors as each shift left little time to sit with students. The staff on Jones ward have come up with a novel solution. When they know it is a student's first week they ensure that the student and the mentor are rostered together on the Wednesday, as there is no elective surgery that afternoon. The student and the mentor then take an extended lunch together of 1 hour, starting at 2 pm once everyone else has returned and there is a good skill mix. As it is planned for in the off-duty, the other staff on shift that day can cover the lunch break without compromising patient care. It is now very rare for students on Jones ward to not have an initial interview in the first week.

It is important that both you and your student are prepared for the initial interview so that you can use the time constructively. Ensure that your student is aware they will need to bring the following to the interview:
- their practice assessment document
- their ongoing achievement record from the previous placement
- any supporting documents, for example, adjustments to be made for disabilities.

In addition, make sure you are fully prepared yourself by reading through the learning outcomes the student will be attempting on the placement in advance of the initial interview.

STAGING THE INITIAL INTERVIEW

The initial interview event will involve a mixture of discussion, writing down information and reading of materials. For this reason it should take place in a location where there is an opportunity to sit comfortably at a table where both you and your student can write. If possible arrange to hold the interview in a quite location away from the general hubbub of the clinical area so that interruptions can be kept to a minimum.

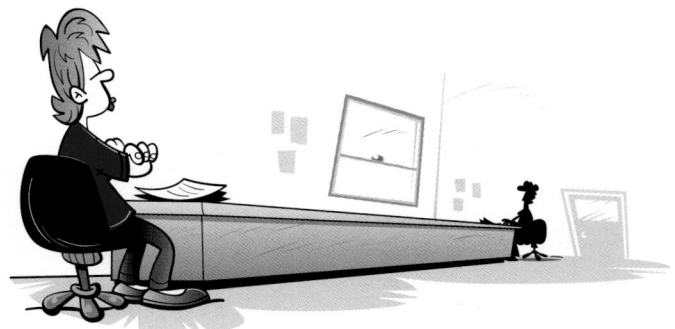

THE INITIAL INTERVIEW...

Nurse's stations, clinic rooms, cars and cafeterias are usually places to avoid for initial interviews. They are either not quiet, not comfortable, or not private (Case study 5.3). Ideally, you should be holding the initial interview in a meeting room, office, teaching room, etc.; somewhere that a door can be closed and noise kept out. If it is acceptable to put a sign on the door to stop interruptions then please do this. Just one hour of protected time at the beginning of a student's placement is worth its weight in gold for both of you.

Case study 5.3 *A mentor speaks about their experience of holding the initial interview*

'We used to conduct the student's initial interview in the patient day room. I'm not sure how that started but it ended up being done there

Continued

Case study 5.3 *A mentor speaks about their experience of holding the initial interview—Cont'd*

out of tradition I think. Anyway, it could not have been a worse possible place. First of all there was no door, so there was very little privacy. It wasn't uncommon for patients and relatives to wander in half way through, wanting to watch TV or drink cups of tea. Eventually someone realized how ridiculous this was and now the students have their initial interviews in the manager's office. They can close the door and have some privacy which is great for everyone.'

BEGINNING THE INTERVIEW

The initial interview is the first formal event that will begin the assessment process during the student's placement. It does not however, need to be held in a formal style, in fact the more relaxed and informal this event is the better for both you and the student. It is formal in the sense that the purpose of the initial interview is to develop an agreed contract of learning and assessment that can be followed and referred to during a student's placement. The initial interview is so important that there is little point in the student being on the placement until it has taken place. Without an initial interview, the student is essentially just working in your clinical area. After the initial interview, the work the student participates in is constantly contributing to their learning and your assessment of their competence.

It's a good idea to have a checklist of issues that need to be covered at the initial interview so that you make the best use of time (Box 5.1). At the very least, the following will need to be discussed:

- learning styles
- reasonable adjustments for disclosed disabilities
- learning outcomes for the placement
- a plan of how learning experiences will be provided
- expectations of competence
- off-duty including confirmation of shift times
- additional learning experiences or goals the student would like to achieve
- an agreement regarding expectations of feedback.

Box 5.1 Best practice for the initial interview

The RCN provides specific advice for conducting an initial interview. Entitled *Guidance for Mentors of Nursing Students and Midwives: An RCN Toolkit*, they recommend the following should be considered during the initial interview

DO find out about the student's stage of training.

DO help the student to form achievable objectives.

DO ask if they have any assignments or assessments.

DO introduce them to the placement learning opportunities.

DO find out if they have any specific anxieties.

DO encourage them to self-assess at every stage.

DO ask if they need any additional support.

RCN (2007) p.11
http://www.rcn.org.uk/__data/assets/pdf_file/0008/78677/002797.pdf

LEARNING STYLES

It is quite common for mentors to begin an initial interview with a student by asking them what they would like to learn. While the intention of this question is well meant, it rarely leads to a satisfactory answer, and can leave both mentor and student floundering for what to say and how to proceed next. A far better way to commence an initial interview is to determine how your student prefers to learn, in otherwise their learning style. There are many different types of learning style categories, however the styles suggested by Honey and Mumford in Box 5.2 tend to be most popular and easiest for most people to relate to. During your initial interview it is very useful to determine what predominant learning style your student may have, as this can make planning of learning experiences far easier for both of you.

DETERMINING LEARNING STYLES

The best way to determine your students preferred learning style is for them to undertake a formal learning style questionnaire, for example the 80-point questionnaire developed by Honey and Mumford. However, from a practical point of view this will just not be possible during an initial interview. You can, however, get some indication of your student's learning style by asking just a few questions (Activity 5.1).

Activity 5.1 Learning styles

It's usually possible to ask a few simple questions to determine your student's preferred learning style. There are some examples of the types of questions you may like to use. If you currently have a student in your practice area you may like to try out some of the questions in this activity.

1. On previous placements have you preferred to observe your mentor demonstrating a task before undertaking the task yourself?

A yes answer may indicate a preference for a reflector or theorist style

2. On previous placements have you preferred to undertake a task rather than observing your mentor doing it first?

A yes answer may indicate a preference for an activist or pragmatist style

3. On previous placements have you tended to ask for explanations of treatment or care before taking part in the treatment or care?

A yes answer may indicate a preference for a reflector or theorist style

4. On previous placements have you tended to ask for explanations of treatment or care after taking part in the treatment or care?

A yes answer may indicate a preference for an activist or pragmatist style

Box 5.2 Honey and Mumford learning styles

Activists

Activists like to take direct action. They are enthusiastic and welcome new challenges and experiences. They are less interested in what has happened in the past or in putting things into a broader context. They are primarily interested in the here and now. They like to have a go, try things out and participate. They like to be the centre of attention.

Reflectors

Reflectors like to think about things in detail without taking any action. They take a thoughtful approach. They are good listeners and prefer to adopt a low profile. They are prepared to read and re-read and will welcome the opportunity to repeat a piece of learning.

Theorists

Theorists like to see how things fall into an overall pattern. They are logical and objective systems people who prefer a sequential approach to problems. They are analytical, pay great attention to detail and tend to be perfectionists.

Pragmatists

Pragmatists like to see how things work in practice. They enjoy experimenting with new ideas. They are practical, down to earth and like to solve problems. They appreciate the opportunity to try out what they have learned are learning.

From Honey and Mumford, 2006, p. 19–20. With permission of Peter Honey Ltd.

> **KEY POINT**
>
> Don't forget to work out your own learning style before asking the student about theirs. This way, you will be able to predict potential clashes in style and plan for how to overcome any challenging situations.

Determining your student's preferred learning style early in the initial interview is invaluable. Don't forget to share what this means with them. For example, if you think that they may be a reflector then share with them that you will try to provide specific opportunities for discussing patient treatment as part of their learning experience. Don't forget to share what your preferred learning style is as potential misunderstandings can be avoided if you are both clear about how you prefer to learn (Case study 5.4).

DEVELOPING ALL LEARNING STYLES

The fact that your student may be predisposed to one particular style of learning does not absolve them from using a range of learning techniques within their placement experiences. In fact, it will be impossible for a student to demonstrate competence in their learning objectives unless they can effectively use a range of learning styles. A reflective or theoretical learning style will be of little use in an emergency situation where thinking fast and accurately on your feet is an imperative. Conversely, an activist or pragmatist learning style will be of little use when needing to carefully look at tables, charts, assessment results from a number of sources before deciding on the best possible course of action. Learning to be a nurse will also mean learning how to use a range of different learning styles appropriate for the different situations you and your student will find yourselves in. There are some examples of how to use different learning styles in Box 5.3.

Case study 5.4 A mentor speaks about a student's learning style

'I remember co-mentoring a student some years ago and I was convinced he was lazy and disinterested. It seemed like every time I suggested doing something new he tried to avoid it and kept asking to read the policy or look in notes. Then I did my mentoring course and we learnt all about learning styles. I suddenly realized that this student wasn't being lazy at all; he was just a theorist in terms of learning style. He obviously felt more comfortable and safe in looking up information before delivering care, especially for something unfamiliar. I guess the fact that I'm an activist meant that I just labelled him as lazy rather than understand where he was coming from.'

Box 5.3 Using different learning styles

Why do I need to be an Activist?

If your least preferred learning style is 'activist' then it is likely that you will not enjoy learning when it involves a new experience or where there are fresh problems to solve. This will create some problems for you in your nurse training as there will be times when action is required and you will need to 'think on your feet'. For example, emergency situations or rapid changes in a patient's clinical condition will require you to make fast and competent decisions as part of a team. This is not the time to spend time thinking through problems or deliberating over the best course of action. Crucially, a part of your learning will be to demonstrate that you can act and react under pressure.

Why do I need to be a Reflector?

If your least preferred learning style is 'reflector' then it is likely that you will not enjoy learning experiences that involve observing problems or thinking through previous experiences. You will probably not enjoy investigating different types of research and ideas and may even feel like these activities are a waste of time. However to demonstrate competence as a nurse you will need to be aware of best practice guidelines and take time to explore alternatives that support evidenced-based practice. For example, new wound care techniques or drug therapies may require changes to your clinical practice.

Why do I need to be a Theorist?

If your least preferred learning style is 'theorist' then it is likely that you will not enjoy spending time over decisions, or lengthy discussions over the best course of action. You may find attention to detail tedious, and become frustrated if you cannot get the answer straight away. However such skills are vital for nurses, whether it is a complex drug calculation or reading carefully through case notes and previous treatment plans, there will be a time when you will need to take the time to carefully think through problems before acting.

Why do I need to be a Pragmatist?

If your least preferred learning style is 'pragmatist' then it is likely that you will not enjoy trying out new techniques, or changing the way you do things. You may not be particularly interested in the consequences of actions or outcomes of events. However 'pragmatic' skills are essential as these activities are strongly linked to evidenced-based practice and being able to adapt and change patient care plans so that the best treatment options are delivered. This includes a range of activities, from monitoring fluid and electrolyte balance to re-evaluating a discharge plan.

From Sharples, 2009, p. 46–47. With permission from Learning Matters.

It is your responsibility to not only develop learning experiences that support a student's learning style, but also develop learning experiences that support the development of a range of styles. This is best done at the initial interview where careful planning of potential learning experiences can be discussed and strengths and weaknesses indentified.

PRACTICE LEARNING OUTCOMES

Once you have gained some insight into your student's preferred learning style, the next stage of the initial interview is to take a very close look at all the learning outcomes for the placement. These will usually be pre-printed in the student's assessment document supplied by the university. The student may have to select from a range of learning outcomes or be required to attempt a set number. Whatever the case it is very important that you confirm from the outset the exact number of outcomes your student will be attempting during the placement. During the placement you will be required to provide learning experiences to support all these outcomes; provide feedback on progress and undertake continual assessment of competence. Both you and your student must be clear from the start the exact outcomes you will be assessing and the learning experiences that need to be catered for.

ONGOING ACHIEVEMENT RECORD

After reviewing your student's learning objectives you should take the time to read and discuss ongoing achievement records from previous placements. This record should highlight student achievements as documented by past mentors, and also any areas of concern or weakness. If there are concerns then you can use this information to plan learning experiences on the current placement. If the student does not have an ongoing achievement record from their previous placement, then you should contact the university immediately. It is an NMC requirement that an ongoing achievement record must be available to you at the beginning of the student placement.

KEY POINT

The only time a student will not have an ongoing achievement record is if they are on the very first practice placement of their first year. At all other times the student is expected to supply you with the record of their previous placement(s).

PLANNING LEARNING EXPERIENCES

The learning outcomes that the student is required to undertake during the placement will largely determine the learning experience you should provide. For example, if the student has a learning outcome related to drug calculations then you will be required to provide learning experiences where drug calculations may be undertaken, for example drug rounds. From this point of view determining a learning plan or contract at the initial interview is a fairly straightforward affair. By discussing openly the learning experiences available and how these will be provided allows both you and your student to discuss expectations on both sides, and troubleshoot foreseeable difficulties.

This should include a frank discussion of difficulties highlighted in the student's ongoing achievement record. There will be a need to negotiate appropriate learning opportunities. For example, you might suggest to your student that they practise drug calculations on the midday drug round rather than the morning round, as this is a quieter time of day and allows more time for discussion and feedback. This is the time to take note also of your student's preferred learning style. If your student is a reflector they may wish to observe you performing calculations and discuss the results before attempting drug calculations themselves. Alternatively, if your student is an activist they may wish to perform drug calculations straight away and discuss these once they have calculated the result. In this case either approach to the learning experience has equal validity, and will ultimately allow you to assess competence.

However, there may well be learning outcomes that require a more fixed approach or learning style. If this is not your student's preferred style of learning then use some time during the initial interview to discuss ways of overcoming this. The main point is that by establishing a learning plan at the initial interview both you and your student will be focused on their learning outcomes and a clear plan for how this can be achieved throughout the placement.

ADDITIONAL LEARNING EXPERIENCES

Apart from the set learning outcomes provided by the university, it may be that your student has some personal learning objectives they would like to achieve during the placement. The initial interview is a great time to discuss these objectives. Remember though, that no matter how keen a student is, they must never exceed the limitations for their current level of competence. As their mentor you are responsible and accountable to monitor this. Just because a student is keen to administer intravenous medications does not mean you should permit this experience.

There will however, be experiences that students can participate in that may not necessarily be covered within their outcomes or highlighted in the assessment document. If in doubt, consult the university regarding what students may and may not participate in. The ongoing achievement record may also point out some experiences that could be included in the student's placement. If they have excelled in a previous experience, then why not set goals that will extend their competence further. Perhaps a previous mentor has indicated that a student has achieved competence in handing over a small number of patients. Why not encourage your student to participate in a ward round during the current placement. Set objectives during the initial interview so that they can be planned for at the same time as the key learning objectives.

DISCLOSURE OF A DISABILITY

It will not be uncommon for a student you are mentoring to disclose to you during the placement that they have a disability. Sadly, some students prefer not to disclose disabilities at all for fear of discrimination. Some students may have experienced a negative response by a mentor following a previous disclosure experience. Some students may not disclose a disability to you until they are some weeks into the placement, perhaps waiting until they have established trust before disclosing this information. Chapter 11 of this book will be dedicated to the subject of mentoring students with disabilities as it requires specific input from a mentor to get it right.

Having said this, the initial interview is a prime opportunity for a student to disclose a disability to you, and you should aim to provide an opportunity for this to be discussed openly and freely. Rather than wait for a student to disclose a disability themselves, it is good practice to raise the subject with all students. You can simply ask if there are any reasonable adjustments or special needs that they want to share with you that will impact on their learning experiences. If a student does not disclose a disability to you at this stage then either they have no disability they are aware of, or they are aware of a disability but are choosing not to disclose. Either way it is their right not to say anything and the initial interview should proceed on this understanding.

If a student does choose to disclose a disability to you at the initial interview then you should feel very privileged. You must have already done quite a bit to gain your student's confidence and respect, they will not have disclosed a disability if they do not feel you can be trusted. Take this as a compliment. Ask your student about the nature of the disability and how this may impact on their learning experience. You can also ask for any supporting material that may have been provided by the university in terms of reasonable adjustments that may be required. Once again please refer to Chapter 11 for specific advice on reasonable adjustments. You can use the information that the student provides to plan their learning experience and make adjustments to the learning plan as required.

KEY POINT

If a student does disclose a disability at initial interview then treat this information with respect. If unsure of how best to support the student seek advice from a lecturer at the university as soon as possible.

EXPECTATIONS OF COMPETENCE

It is virtually impossible to develop a learning plan without discussing expectations of competence with your student. Remember that they are undertaking the placement not only for learning experiences to be provided, but also to determine their competence reflected in the learning outcomes. As the assessor of competence, you must be confident about your expectations of competence for each learning objective from the outset. You must share and discuss these expectations with your student when developing each learning plan. It is very helpful if you not only document the learning plan in their assessment document, but also make a note of what you will be expecting in order to assess the outcome as achieved. Remember that your expectations of competence should include equal measures of knowledge, skill and professionalism. It is worthwhile spelling out from the beginning exactly what these expectations are for each learning outcome, and what you will be looking for in order to sign them off as having been achieved.

The initial interview is no time to be vague or confuse a student with ambiguous statements. Your student deserves to know what is expected of them so that they can have some clear goals to aim towards (Activity 5.2). Your student should also be made aware that their assessment will be based on evidence from a wide variety of sources, and that while you will be the assessor, other mentors and registered nurses will contribute to the overall assessment of competence.

Activity 5.2 Planning a learning scenario

Have a go at planning a learning experience. Start by choosing a learning objective that is commonly attempted by students in your area. Next write a quick plan of the learning experiences this will involve. Finish the plan by writing your expectations of competence. Here is an example to get you started.

Learning outcome	Learning plan	Evidence of competence
Perform drug calculations accurately	Every shift the student will practise at least three drug calculations on the midday drug round.	Skill – Accuracy of all drug calculations. Knowledge – Knows all calculation formulas. Professionalism – Demonstrates accountability in double checking all drug calculations.

After deciding on a learning plan and expectations of competence it is very important that you document all these considerations in the student's practice assessment document (PAD). Not only does this provide the evidence of what has been discussed, it also provides a very clear benchmark of what should take place during the placement. If your student happens to work alongside a co-mentor during the placement they will be able to show the learning plan developed at the initial interview as a guide for learning in your absence. Documentary evidence of the learning plan developed at the initial interview will also provide the basis for feedback throughout the placement. Both you and your student will be able to refer to the agreement made at the initial interview as a basis by which to discuss progress and achievement of objectives.

KEY POINT

While the students in your clinical area may change, the learning outcomes students attempt will probably stay the same. Why not agree within your team the types of experiences suitable and the expectations of competence for each outcome. In this way students will be provided with a good range of experiences and are more likely to be assessed fairly by all mentors.

PLANNING THE OFF-DUTY

While the development of a learning plan and expectations of competence are the focus of the initial interview, there are additional elements to this event which must not be forgotten. No matter how good your learning plan is, it will be a failure unless you and your student spend the majority of their placement working together. As the main mentor you must make a commitment to ensuring that the student spends enough time with you to enable a fair and accurate assessment of their competence (Case study 5.5). In order to achieve this goal you should aim to provide the student with the same off-duty as yourself. If there are days or nights when this is not possible then arrange a co-mentor for the student, someone that can follow-up on progress on your behalf and also provide clear and accurate feedback. This person will need to be briefed on the learning plan and expectations of competence also – all the more reason to write this down at the initial interview.

Case study 5.5 Working with a student

Kate is an experienced mentor who has learnt the value of working consistently with her student. When she is allocated a student by her manager her first step is to check her own off-duty to check that she does not have any holidays booked during the student's placement. If this does happen she asks her manager to re-allocate the student to another mentor. Once Kate has confirmed that she will be available for the whole of the placement she makes sure that the student is allocated the same shifts as herself. Kate makes sure her student receives this rota before the placement commences, usually at the pre-placement visit. By following these very easy steps Kate ensures she will be able to provide the best possible learning experiences and feedback throughout the placement.

It is crucial that you make time in the initial interview to clarify the off-duty with your student, and ascertain if there will be any difficulties for them following your work rota. If there are difficulties in terms of family or work commitments then these must be highlighted and if any concerns discussed with the university.

KEY POINT

It will be impossible to undertake a continual assessment of your student's progress unless you spend the majority of their placement working together. Use the initial interview to plan the off-duty to maximize your opportunity to assess student competence.

SCHEDULING FEEDBACK

The completion of the initial interview will mark the beginning of the assessment phase during the student's clinical placement. For this reason it is very important to negotiate with your student a schedule of feedback during the placement experience. You should aim to discuss the frequency of feedback and what will be covered during feedback. Chapter 6 of this book will look specifically at feedback so we won't go into too much detail just now. However, it is important that you discuss what your student can expect from you in terms of feedback during the placement at the initial interview. If you are planning on providing informal feedback then the student should be prepared for this. In addition, you should also plan for formal feedback events, specifically the midpoint interview. If possible, try to agree the date of the midpoint interview with your student at the end of the initial interview. It can then be a set event that you both plan for and can prepare for in advance.

PERSONALITY CLASHES

Like all human relationships, clashes of personality between a student and a mentor can occur. Personality clashes are less likely if you are prepared for the student and the placement gets off to a good start for both of you. The risk of personality clashes can also be reduced if there is clear and friendly communication between you and your student early in the placement, and the initial interview is the ideal time to cement a positive working relationship. Remember that your role in the mentor/student relationship is to provide learning experiences and to undertake a fair and accurate assessment of competence. You are required to be friendly towards your student; however do not make the mistake of wishing to become friends. Blurring the line between mentor and friend will only result in role confusion and can lead to students feeling betrayed, especially in feedback situations.

UNDERSTANDING THE DOCUMENTATION

At the end of the initial interview you should clarify with your student how the documentation within the PAD will be completed. In Chapter 4 we identified the key elements of a PAD; however changes can take place and you must make sure you are familiar with the one being used for each placement. It is not uncommon for PADs to vary slightly between first-, second- and third-year students so don't assume they are all the same.

ACCESS TO THE PAD

You should also ensure that your student is clear regarding when you will need to see the PAD after the initial interview. If you want it available daily so you can review learning outcomes then make this clear. If your student is concerned regarding how to keep the document safe then offer them a locked cupboard or room if you have not already done so. While these may seem small issues they can easily be the source of controversy and disharmony if not clarified from the outset.

CONTACT NUMBERS

It is often useful to have a student's contact details: for example, phone number or email, so you can contact them if needed during the placement. The student does not have to provide you with these as it is personal information; however, they may do so if they wish. Discuss contact details with the student at the initial interview, and clarify the situations that you will contact them under. This may include an unplanned change to the shift pattern of if you are concerned about unexplained non-attendance. You will need to make it clear that you will keep their details for the placement period only, and not disclose them to others.

KEY POINT

Contact details of students must be kept in a confidential place and never disclosed to third parties. If a student does not wish to disclose their private contact details then ensure you are aware how to contact them via the university.

MAKING THE MOST OF THE INITIAL INTERVIEW

The initial interview is your best opportunity to establish very clearly with the student that you will be taking on the role of mentor and assessor during the placement. It is your chance to clarify exactly what they can expect from you in this role and to form a positive working relationship. It will take effort, commitment and planning to ensure that this becomes a reality. If you leave the initial interview to chance you run the risk of conducting it in a rush or conducting it too late in the placement to be of benefit. To avoid this you will need to prepare for and schedule the initial interview as a distinct event during the student's first week of placement. You will also need the support of your colleagues to ensure the event is not interrupted. However, time spent at this stage will not be wasted, and can prevent potential problems from occurring later in the placement. The initial interview allows you and your student to clarify the nature of your relationship and set clear boundaries and expectations that will form the basis of all future placement decisions.

 TOP TIPS

- Try to schedule a student's initial interview into the planned off-duty for the first week. Ask your colleagues to cover your work so the time can be ring-fenced.
- Explore your own learning style as this will help you to understand similarities and differences in how you and your student approach learning.
- Use the ongoing achievement record to plan learning experiences with the student. In this way you will be able to acknowledge the student's strengths and provide a focused plan for developing weaknesses.
- Don't try to become 'friends' with a student. Use a friendly approach but remember to stay professional and objective.

References

Honey P, Mumford A (2006) *The Learning Styles Questionnaire – 80 Point Item*. Peter Honey Publications, Maidenhead.

Sharples K (2009) *Learning to Learn in Nursing Practice*. Learning Matters, Exeter.

CHAPTER 6

GIVING FEEDBACK

Chapter Aims

The purpose of this chapter is to assist you with understanding the role of feedback in relation to the assessment process and the student learning experience. After reading this chapter you will be able to:

- Identify the key aspects of verbal and written feedback.
- Understand the relevance of the feedback sandwich in facilitating learning.
- Consider the professional accountability and responsibility in delivering feedback.
- Develop your competence and confidence for feedback experiences.

FEEDBACK

For many mentors, giving feedback to students is one of the biggest challenges and probably the most difficult aspects of their role. It is not uncommon for even experienced mentors to be nervous about giving a student feedback regarding their performance, particularly when the feedback is not positive. In fact, some mentors are so reluctant to give feedback to students that they avoid doing it at all. It can be very tempting to delay or avoid evaluation meetings with students for fear of a negative response or over-reaction to criticism. In addition, the pressure of the clinical environment, for example staffing levels or very busy shifts can also impact on the delivery of feedback. This is highly problematic, as providing time for reflection, giving feedback, monitoring and documenting a student's progress are all vital if the assessment process is to be followed and the student is to be given every opportunity to improve. If feedback has not been consistent throughout the placement, students may be confused regarding the decisions you are making related to their learning outcomes, and you may find you lack the evidence to support your decisions. It is also important to realize that if you don't provide your student with feedback you will not be meeting the standards expected by the NMC in relation to mentorship, which has serious professional implications.

PREVIOUS EXPERIENCE OF FEEDBACK

If you have already had experience of giving feedback to a student it is likely that you will have had a mix of experiences; some of these may have been positive, while others may have been less than satisfactory. There will always be reasons for these different experiences; however they can only be properly analysed by taking a step back and reflecting objectively on each experience. Understanding the circumstances surrounding each of the different types of feedback events you have experienced can provide a useful guide in understanding where improvements are needed (Activity 6.1).

Feedback requires a number of factors to be in place to be effective. It takes both confidence and skill to deliver feedback in a way that is helpful to the student. Feedback also needs to take place in the right environment with sufficient time to discuss any issues of concern or areas for further development. If any of these elements are lacking then it is quite possible that your feedback experience will be unsatisfactory. Take a look at the key areas of each feedback situation that you reflected on in Activity 6.1. In terms of your negative experience, did you have sufficient knowledge or skill in relation to giving feedback? Was the environment right and did you have sufficient time? If the answer is no to any of these questions then this probably explains why the event was unsatisfactory. Now look at the positive event. What particular knowledge, skills or resources made the difference here? Hopefully you can start to see that the difference in each event is not you personally; it is the combination of circumstances, skills and knowledge that together can separate positive and negative feedback experiences.

Activity 6.1 Reflecting on previous experiences of giving feedback

Reflect on one feedback situation that you feel went particularly well. Now make some brief notes about why you feel the situation went well. For example, you might like to comment about the environment, the stage of the assessment, what you discussed with the student.

Now reflect on a feedback experience that was unsatisfactory and use the same process to make some brief notes about what took place. Try to focus on the factors that you feel contributed to the negative feedback experience.

PREPARATION FOR FEEDBACK

Without any doubt the preparation of mentors for delivering effective feedback to students is vital and if you have not been well prepared for this event it is likely to become either chaotic or very uncomfortable. If you are lacking the confidence and skill to give fair and accurate feedback, then you are certainly not alone. While feedback is a vital component of fair and accurate assessment, you must also ensure that vulnerable students are protected and their self-esteem is not damaged as a result of your feedback. As a result feedback often becomes a delicate balancing act between protecting a student's feelings and being honest. If you are not prepared or not confident in how to do this a feedback situation can be very daunting indeed. In order to address these issues we must take a fresh look at feedback; what it is, what it isn't; and most importantly, how to get it right.

ASSESSMENT AND FEEDBACK

The assessment of pre-registration students can best be described as a 'process', with regular feedback to students being an integral aspect of this process. You cannot decide to 'opt out' of providing feedback as the process then falters. If you fail to provide a student with feedback then you are not only failing to fulfil your professional role as a mentor but you are also failing in your obligation to the student. Students value feedback and define this as an attribute of a 'good' mentor (see Case study 6.1), whereas a mentor who gives no feedback or delivers it in a way that is unhelpful to the student will be poorly evaluated by a student. So let's look at feedback in more detail.

WHAT IS FEEDBACK?

Feedback is the main way that you will provide a student with a review of their performance during a practice placement. It is both opinion based and a judgement. It is for this reason that many mentors do not like giving feedback. They either feel uncomfortable providing an opinion or in making a judgement about a student's performance. However, your primary role as a mentor is to assess students, and to do this you must form both an opinion and make a judgement regarding your student's competence. Remember though that although feedback is based on a judgement of student competence, this competence should always be related to the learning outcomes the student is trying to achieve. Your role is not to

You should not expect that students will recognize their mistakes and take appropriate action without some feedback from you. No matter how obvious it may seem to you, a student will rarely take action to rectify a problem unless you have discussed this with them and explored how to improve their performance. So, feedback must be clear, and feedback must be timely.

KEY POINT

Students rely on honest feedback to identify their progress during the placement. They expect that if there are concerns about their progress then they will be informed of this. Unless students hear otherwise, they will assume that there are no problems with their competence.

WHEN SHOULD I GIVE FEEDBACK?

We've already established that students expect feedback. They want to hear from you how they are performing. Keeping this in mind you will need to provide your student with feedback from the very beginning of their placement. While it is up to you as to how often and when you provide feedback to a student during their placement, it is worth remembering that the NMC expects that you will provide feedback to a student as often as it is needed to guide performance.

As an essential aspect of formative assessment, feedback can help students to rate their clinical performance more realistically. If students are not reaching a competent standard then feedback should be more frequent to provide opportunities to develop and improve. However, you do need to take care to ensure that you are not overdoing your feedback, as students may feel threatened by this. It is essential therefore that you have a clear understanding of the different types of feedback that you will give throughout a student's placement.

INFORMAL FEEDBACK

Informal feedback can occur any time throughout a clinical placement and is usually given in response to a specific event. It can happen at any time and is generally unplanned. It may take place on-the-spot or as an informal conversation some time after an event or situation occurs in practice. In general, the earlier in a placement that informal feedback becomes routine between a mentor and student the better. Both you and your student will benefit from establishing frequent and spontaneous lines of communication. Insufficient feedback can have a negative impact on the student learning experience, resulting in increased anxiety and insecurity during clinical placement. However, if feedback is regularly given then it can be used to support the student's learning and provide great opportunities for reflection.

Mentors also benefit from providing students with regular feedback, as you will gain confidence in discussing your student's progress with them. You may find that some students request continual feedback, and you may have to put some limitations on this. If your student does require frequent feedback then you may choose to plan ahead for specific time periods where this may be possible. It's also a good idea to put a time limit on your discussions to ensure the time used is focused.

Keep in mind that either you or your student can instigate feedback. You may volunteer feedback, or your student may request feedback from you. However it is often rare for a student to actually say 'Can I have some feedback?'. Students will often request feedback by asking for a specific comment regarding a clinical situation in which they have been involved. For example, they may request feedback by asking 'Was that OK?' or 'How did I do?' Try to seize these opportunities when students request feedback to provide them with an honest and useful answer. If they broach the subject then they want to hear your answer and this is a great time to give accurate feedback and also to further probe the student's understanding of what has been happening. However, where a student is reluctant to receive feedback it is important to ensure that your feedback relates to the student's learning outcomes and is non-threatening.

KEY POINT

Informal feedback is flexible. It can range from immediate on-the-spot feedback, or be delivered as a summary of the student's performance at the end of the day. Feedback should take place as close to an event as possible to ensure relevance and accuracy of reflection.

FORMAL FEEDBACK

Formal feedback is a planned event and is usually delivered at predetermined stages of the clinical placement, namely, the initial interview, midpoint review and final assessment. It should be structured and ideally be conducted in a quiet area away from the noise and distraction of the practice environment. It is very important that you ensure privacy and

Box 6.1 Checklist for formal feedback

Set the time and date with your student for all formal feedback.	☐
Ensure the student has plenty of opportunity to prepare for it.	☐
Tell your student what you would like to discuss during the interview.	☐
Ask your student what they would like to discuss.	☐
Agree what you will discuss.	☐

allow adequate time for what you say to be digested and understood by the student. Formal feedback can be more challenging than informal feedback. Some mentors find it particularly difficult to instigate and deliver feedback in a formal setting, mainly due to the strong emotional dimension of the interaction. You should also remember that students may also feel vulnerable when receiving feedback as this is your opinion of their performance, and will be directly related to the final decision you make for the placement learning outcomes.

For this reason formal feedback events should never be 'sprung' on a student without prior warning. What you are going to say should always be planned in order to make the best use of the time. If you do not plan what you are going to say during feedback then there may be inconsistencies between what you say and what others have said during the placement, which will only increase student insecurity and anxiety. Your student also needs time to prepare themselves for the feedback event. Students who are not given sufficient warning of a formal interview may feel quite intimidated, and reluctant to voice their opinions or concerns. A lack of two-way interaction will jeopardize the interaction needed for insight and development. Keep in mind that if your student enters a formal interview feeling negative for any reason then the time you spend with them will be of little benefit. In Box 6.1 there are some suggested elements to help you prepare for a formal feedback situation.

DELIVERING FEEDBACK

Many mentors fall into the trap of only delivering feedback when there is a concern regarding a student's performance. Students who are achieving all outcomes may miss out on feedback because they are seen to be 'doing OK'. It is quite common to find mentors who associate feedback with poor performance, rather than as a tool to encourage achievement. Typically, it is the informal feedback that students will be denied if they are producing a satisfactory performance. However, there is great value in delivering simple and frequent praise for students who are achieving. Not only is this a great boost to self-esteem but it will also make your overall assessment more credible if you make it obvious that you are reviewing the student's performance as a whole rather than picking on isolated events. Don't ever forget that a little praise goes a long way.

CLEAR FEEDBACK

Regardless of what type of feedback you are giving, remember that it must be clear and unambiguous. Too little information and the student may be unsure of what it is you are saying, what is required of them or how this relates to their learning outcomes. When information is withheld, then feedback becomes a superficial exercise and will be of little value to a student. If feedback includes too much information the student may feel overwhelmed, taking in little of what you have actually said. Feedback should always include examples from practice and should also include specific targets and standards. If your feedback is not clear then ultimately your student may lack direction. If you fail to link your feedback with events that have taken place during the placement then the student may be confused regarding their performance (Case study 6.3).

Case study 6.3 A student speaks of her experience of feedback

'When I was in my second year my mentor called me into the office one day and started to talk to me about the need to communicate with the Health Care Assistants on the ward. After about 5 minutes of her explaining all about the role of Health Care Assistants she asked me how I felt and I remember giving some response about how the information had been useful and then we walked out together. I remember thinking that it was really nice to have a one on one teaching session with my mentor. About a week later I had my final interview and she started referring to the 'feedback' she had given me about delegating care, and how I hadn't really improved. I told her I couldn't remember any feedback on that, and then, out of the blue she explained that the teaching session was actually her feedback on something I wasn't achieving. I was so upset, if only she had been clear I would have been able to ask questions about what to do. I realize now that I missed out on getting help to improve because she was too nervous to actually be honest about the issue.'

FEEDBACK ABOUT CONCERNS

If you are giving feedback for the purpose of improving student performance you must ensure that you are clear about the problem, a student will not change behaviour if they do not know what needs to be corrected. Therefore you cannot and must not rely on assumptions or inferences to deliver feedback. Your failure to be honest about performance problems may subsequently lead to confrontation as students may interpret your poor feedback as inconsistent and dishonest. Such is the importance of honesty in delivering feedback that some students have rated this element as the number one characteristic of a mentor. For this reason it is vital that once feedback has been delivered that you clarify what has been said in order to rectify any misconceptions. You should remember that the feedback given may not always be the same as the feedback received, so encourage students to reflect on your feedback and outline their interpretation of its content.

KEY POINT

Feedback must always be honest and consistent. You must ensure that your student understands the feedback you have given, and how the feedback related to their learning outcomes.

CONSTRUCTIVE FEEDBACK

A lack of clarity in feedback can have a detrimental effect on the student–mentor relationship and can compromise the self-esteem of the mentor and the student. You must therefore ensure that the feedback you give is always constructive, whether it is delivered informally or formally. Constructive feedback is:
- objective
- non-judgemental
- based on specific evidence
- motivating
- encourages discussion
- allows for a positive course to be set for the future
- boosts student confidence
- encourages future learning.

As a mentor you will also benefit from providing feedback to students through sharing practice, enhancing learning and allowing students the opportunity to reflect on their practice. Spontaneous feedback is especially valuable as it provides a platform for a student to undertake self-reflection of their performance and gives you valuable insight into the student's perception of their own ability. For this reason self-reflection should be encouraged in feedback situations. The student's self-reflection should also provide opportunities for a clear discussion on strengths and weaknesses, and help students to plan further learning experiences. Without clarity of feedback, students risk engaging in reflective exercises that are not related to the development of clinical competence and as a result may miss potential learning experiences.

FEEDBACK AND SELF-ESTEEM

While you may deliver feedback in an honest and encouraging way this will not always ensure that a student responds positively to your feedback. Although it is reasonable to assume that honesty is important, a student may not interpret the feedback as encouraging if they are vulnerable due to low self-esteem. In fact students with low self-esteem may have a fear of negative evaluation and avoid feedback situations as a way of coping. While students with high self-esteem may view feedback as an opportunity to improve, those with low self-esteem may see it as threatening and therefore the feedback needs to be carefully handled.

For this reason you must always ensure that you deliver feedback in positive terms in order to maintain or improve self-esteem. This approach will be fairly simple when providing praise for students who are performing well and reaching a high standard; however it creates difficulties when feedback is required to point out errors or poor performance. As there is always a tendency for students with low self-esteem to take any comment as an indictment of themselves, feedback must always be related to the student's work performance and never based on the character of the student.

> **KEY POINT**
>
> The self-esteem of students must be taken into account when delivering feedback. Feedback should be directly related to specific learning outcomes and not directed towards personal attributes or a student's character.

THE FEEDBACK SANDWICH

The feedback sandwich is usually the best and fairest way of delivering both formal and informal feedback. It should consist of one specific area for improvement 'sandwiched' between two specific praises (Case study 6.4). It is a particularly useful technique when giving feedback to students with low self-esteem, as, when used correctly, it begins and ends with positive statements. In fact a well-timed, well-targeted and well-constructed feedback sandwich will:

- encourage student learning
- motivate future learning
- reduce confusion
- improve self-esteem
- value the student's contribution to their learning.

Case study 6.4 *Delivering a feedback sandwich*

Kevin is undertaking a placement in a care of the elderly ward. In his first week his mentor has noticed that he is very keen to involve himself in all aspects of patient care, but seems to avoid situations where he is required to deliver care to one particular patient who is confused and has frequent outbursts of verbal aggression. His mentor decides to use a feedback sandwich to open up a discussion on Kevin's feelings related to this patient.

Praise

'Hi Kevin, I just wanted to say well done on your first week here, I'm really pleased with how keen you are to care for the patients. You're making really good progress in your learning outcomes related to dignity and respect, so well done.'

Concern

'I'm sorry about Mr Jones' verbal aggression. I could see by your reaction on Tuesday when he was yelling that you felt uncomfortable talking with him.'

Praise

'I'd like to work with you on that, as I have seen how much potential you have in communicating with most patients. How would you feel about us developing a plan to communicate with Mr Jones so that you can achieve that outcome?'

KEY POINT

The feedback sandwich is the best way to deliver feedback constructively. It can correct practice while maintaining a student's self-esteem.

DOCUMENTING FEEDBACK

Without any question, the one area that most mentors consistently find difficult is documenting feedback. In particular, mentors often struggle with the wording of written feedback and are concerned with the fact that what they write is permanently recorded in the student's assessment document. Some students may discourage their mentors from documenting feedback, especially in situations where there is a need for change and improvement in performance. Yet we know that without a written record of an event there is no evidence to support what has been done or said. The *Standards to Support Learning and Assessment in Practice* (NMC, 2008) state clearly the position of the NMC in relation to written feedback.

> *The NMC considers it important that mentors have an audit trail to support their decisions. Throughout a placement where a critical decision on progress is to be made the mentor should ensure that regular feedback is given to the student and that records are kept of guidance given.*
>
> *(NMC, 2008, p. 34)*

The professional obligation here is quite clear. As a registered nurse you are accountable and responsible to the NMC for the assessment decision you make about a student nurse. You must therefore ensure that your written report provides clear and accurate records of events during the student's practice placement. The clearer and more specific your documentation is, the more clarity there will be to support the steps you have taken in the assessment process. Documented feedback will contribute to the 'audit trail' within the practice placement and provide evidence that supports your decision to pass or fail a student on their learning outcomes. You are therefore professionally obligated to document the feedback you give to a student as this will provide the evidence to support the assessment process and your assessment decision.

WHAT DO I WRITE?

Your documentation of feedback needs to be both fair and accurate. It must also reflect any verbal discussions that you have had with your student. It is important that you write clear and accurate notes about any verbal feedback you have given and stick to the facts of what was said, not adding in any information that was not discussed. Documented feedback must not be kept from the student or written in secret, nor should it ever appear in notes or letters that do not form the assessment documentation. If you do this the student will interpret this as collaborating against them rather than working with them.

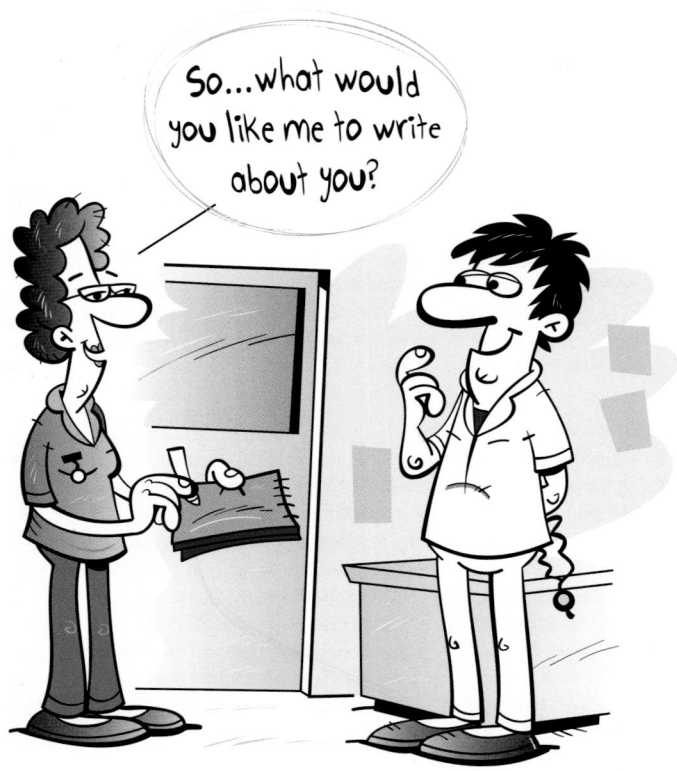

You must resist the temptation to dilute your written feedback in order to spare a student's feelings as this will result in an inaccurate recording of events. In fact, a discrepancy between what is said and what is written only increases student anxiety, as a non-specific report can seriously undermine student confidence. Written feedback should also be dated and signed by you and the student as it often forms the basis of a learning contract or action plan. You may find it helpful to use the feedback sandwich for your written documentation as this will ensure that you are consistent in your approach and can aid in setting specific standards and targets. In addition, students can use your documentation of feedback to discuss their learning needs with other staff in your clinical area and lecturers from the university.

WHERE DO I WRITE?

Written feedback should be recorded within the practice assessment document (PAD) that the university has provided for you. There will generally be a section within the PAD allocated for mentors to record their feedback. This will probably be highlighted within or following initial, midpoint and end interviews. However, additional documentation is always welcomed by the universities and it is worth finding out where in the assessment document you should write this. It may be in the form of an action plan, ongoing record of achievement, or a general report section. The amount you write is generally up to you however it should be enough to ensure that your concerns or assessment decisions are fully explained and that your student is aware of what is required of them for improvement.

KEY POINT

All feedback must be recorded in the student's assessment document. Remember that if it isn't written down, there will be no evidence of the feedback that you have provided.

DIFFICULT FEEDBACK

There may be times as a mentor when you are faced with a situation where you must give a student very difficult feedback. The common areas where feedback may be the most difficult include:

- feedback that confirms a student has failed an element or elements of practice learning outcomes

- students with very poor self-esteem who are not making satisfactory progress
- students who are unable to accept limitations in their competence.

In such situations you would be well advised to seek help in delivering the feedback. In each situation the best person to provide support must be decided upon at the time, as there are many variables to consider. For example, in some situations another mentor in the practice area may be considered the best alternative, especially if the student has built a rapport with this person. However, there is the risk with this approach that a student may consider that 'everyone' in the practice area is ganging up on them.

Link lecturers may also be consulted by mentors for difficult feedback situations, and sometimes a student may appreciate having a university lecturer present for support (Case study 6.5). At other times students may perceive this action as 'bringing in the big guns' and be even more intimidated by this outcome.

Case study 6.5 *A link lecturer speaks of a difficult feedback situation*

'I remember supporting a mentor who was very apprehensive about providing feedback for a student at the final interview. She was so nervous she was physically shaking. The student had tried very hard during the placement but had just not achieved three of her learning outcomes. She had been supported throughout; however, the mentor was still very apprehensive about discussing the final result. As their conversation progressed the student became quite upset and began to cry. It was a very difficult situation for this mentor as she was obviously upset herself. I realized that the student somehow thought that the non-achievement of her outcomes signalled the end of her training. I was so glad I was there, as I was able to explain that this was not correct, she would simply be given a further placement to achieve the outcomes. It became clear that neither the mentor nor student were aware of this fact. Once the option of a further placement became clear the atmosphere in the room changed immediately. If I had not been there I just don't know what the outcome would have been.'

The key to delivering difficult feedback is to access the most appropriate support and then deliver the feedback as professionally as possible. Avoiding difficult feedback is not, and will never be, the solution.

DOCUMENTING THE ONGOING ACHIEVEMENT RECORD

It is an NMC requirement that a record of a student's progress be made available from one placement to the next. Ideally this will be documented by the primary mentor at the conclusion of the placement, following the final interview. This record should provide a brief summary of the placement and clearly identify learning outcomes the student has achieved and also record any areas that require development in subsequent placements.

The ongoing achievement record should not contain any information that has not been discussed with the student during the placement; rather it should be a summary of events during the placement. This information will be invaluable to the student and subsequent mentors to chart the student's progress and will help identify any areas that require particular development plans on future placements. Without this information the student's progress through their learning experiences will be compromised and it denies them the considerable benefits of a continual and focused learning experience.

FAIR AND HONEST FEEDBACK

Feedback is an essential aspect of the student assessment process. Accurate verbal and written feedback is essential in order to encourage students to reflect on their learning and provides an opportunity to identify how they can improve their performance. In addition, appropriate feedback supports the assessment process and your assessment decision. At all times, whether written or verbal your feedback must be fair and honest. The NMC makes it quite clear that mentors are professionally obligated to provide students with fair and timely feedback. The feedback sandwich is the most judicious and fair way of delivering both formal and informal feedback. This is particular relevant for students with low self-esteem who are at risk of perceiving feedback as a personal attack. For this reason feedback must be well timed, well targeted and well said in order to direct growth, to motivate and to offer relief from confusion.

TOP TIPS

- Try to set a 'feedback schedule' at the beginning of the placement to ensure you habitually deliver it and the student comes to expect it.
- Identify students who are vulnerable or display low self-esteem and moderate your feedback accordingly.
- Use the feedback sandwich every time you deliver feedback.
- Remember that if feedback isn't written down it didn't happen.

Reference

Nursing and Midwifery Council (2008) *Standards to Support Learning and Assessment in Practice: NMC Standards for Mentors, Practice Teachers and Teachers*. NMC, London, available from http://www.nmc-uk.org.

CHAPTER 7

THE MIDPOINT INTERVIEW

Chapter Aims

The purpose of this chapter is to explore the nature and function of the midpoint interview. After reading the chapter you will be able to:

- Explain the purpose of the midpoint interview.
- Identify the essential components of a successful midpoint interview.
- Successfully conduct a midpoint interview.

WHAT IS THE PURPOSE OF THE MIDPOINT INTERVIEW?

In Chapter 6 we discussed the importance of giving feedback to your student on the progress they are making towards achieving their learning outcomes. The chapter established that feedback is essential in helping the student to achieve competence. We also identified that feedback can be given both informally and formally. In this chapter, we will focus on one of the specific times when formal feedback, based on detailed assessment of progress, is given, that is, the midpoint interview.

The main purpose of the midpoint interview is to discuss with your student their progress and performance to date, identify strengths and weaknesses, outcomes achieved and those areas where further development is needed. The midpoint interview is a key step in the assessment process, allowing both you and your student the chance to look back on what they have achieved during the preceding weeks, and to plan for what still needs to be done. At this stage, both you and your student should have a clear idea of whether or not the required level of performance is likely to be achieved within the time remaining.

Chapter 6 also highlighted how you as a mentor will be continuously assessing your student's level of competence, providing guidance, support and regular feedback to help your student achieve their outcomes. During this process, you will be recording your observations and informal discussions within the practice assessment document. In essence you will be continually monitoring your student's progress. At some point however, you will need to take stock of how far you and your student have come on the learning journey. You will both need to take 'time out' to review progress made, reflect on the good bits and the not so good bits of the placement so far and plan for the 'second half'. The midpoint interview represents half time. It is a time to evaluate, regroup and refocus. It is a time to review the initial learning plan and decide whether this has been effective. It is the time to ask questions such as:

- Have the goals you set at the initial interview been achieved?
- Have the different aspects of the learning plan worked in the way they were designed to?
- Were any changes made to the plan and why?
- What still needs to be done in order to achieve the desired goals?
- What are you and your student going to do now to get to where they need to be?

The midpoint interview is a time for you to re-energize, re-motivate and spur the student on to bigger and better things in the second half of the practice placement.

PURPOSE OF THE MIDPOINT INTERVIEW

Although the midpoint interview is a formal step in the assessment process, it is a formative rather than a summative component of assessment. The purpose of the midpoint interview is to identify and provide information that you can effectively use to improve your student's learning rather than to test whether the specific learning outcomes have been achieved. At the midpoint interview, you are measuring how far your student has progressed towards achieving the set goals, identifying their successes and where they may be having trouble. You can then use this information to make necessary adjustments to their learning plan, such as changing your style of mentoring, identifying and/or offering alternative or further opportunities for practice. The feedback you give as part of the midpoint interview should help your student become aware of any gaps that exist between their desired goal and their current knowledge, understanding or skills and guide them through the actions necessary to achieve that goal. The purpose of formative feedback is to enhance learning not to pass judgement. The key function of the midpoint interview therefore is to inform both you and your learner about what has already been learnt and what has still to be achieved.

WHEN SHOULD THE INTERVIEW TAKE PLACE?

Mentoring like all processes requires that each stage is completed at the proper time and in the proper manner if the whole system is to work successfully. A delay in any stage, skipping of any of the stages, or focusing too much on a single stage will lead to confusion and poor results. It is therefore important that the midpoint interview is carried out at an appropriate point in the student's placement. So when should you carry out the midpoint interview? Case study 7.1 provides a possible midpoint interview scenario.

There are clearly a number of concerns arising from this encounter but for the time being let's consider the timing of this meeting. Gina has started her sixth week of an eight-week placement. Her mentor Carol has therefore had five weeks to monitor her progress, so in this respect should have a clear picture of Gina's capabilities and areas requiring improvement. However, Gina has less than three weeks of her placement left. What happens if Carol decides Gina is not making adequate progress towards achieving the set learning outcomes? What if she identifies that Gina is struggling in several areas? Gina has less than three weeks left to work on any weak areas. Is this sufficient time for Gina to have the opportunity to work on these areas? If the purpose of mentoring is to facilitate learning and development, it is crucial that formative assessment is timely (try Activity 7.1).

Case study 7.1 Gina's midpoint interview

It is Gina's sixth week of an eight-week placement to Disraeli ward. She has asked to see her mentor Carol.

Carol 'Oh hi, erm, Gina? You said you wanted to see me! I've got a few minutes so what is it you want to see me about?'

Gina 'We've got to sign something off in my practice book.'

Carol 'Oh, right!'

Gina 'I haven't seen you since my initial interview. There is something in my book you have to sign off.'

Carol 'Do you know where it is?' (Takes the book from Gina.)

Gina 'It's nothing much. You just need to sign to say how I'm getting on.'

Carol 'Oh yes! The midpoint interview'. (Reading from the practice book) 'It says here this should take place during weeks three and four. How long have you been here now?'

Gina 'Nearly six weeks!'

Carol 'Oh dear! A bit late aren't we? Ah well, it doesn't matter, we can get something written down!'

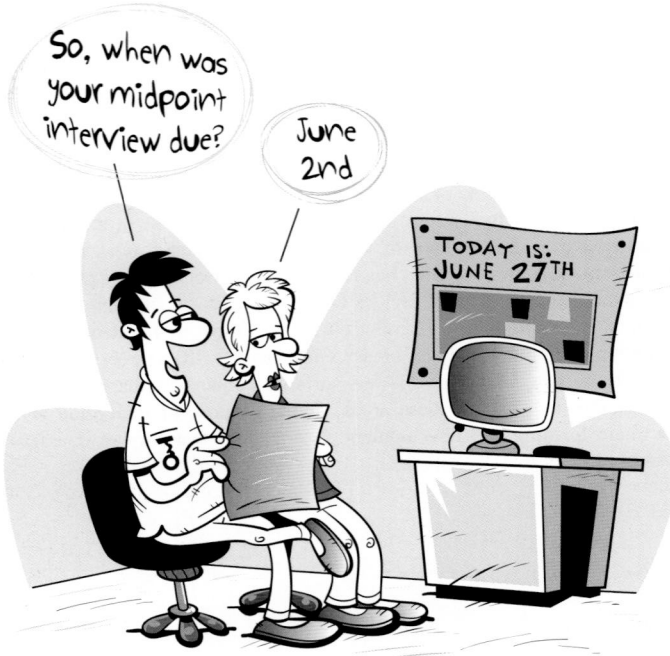

The midpoint interview therefore needs to take place at a point in the student's placement that will allow plenty of time and opportunity for him/her to address any weaknesses. There has to be time for the student

Activity 7.1 Midpoint interviews in your area

If possible, try to complete a quick audit of when midpoint interviews are generally carried out in your clinical area. Try to find the data regarding the assessment process of some past (or present) students in your clinical area. For each student try to identify the following:
1. In which week should the midpoint interview have taken place?
2. In which week did the midpoint interview take place?
Try to include as many students as possible in your sample so you can get an accurate idea of the trends for your practice area.

to participate in the necessary learning experiences, practise and refine skills if they are to gain competence. The ideal therefore is to time the midpoint interview at a point in the placement where progress can be properly established and advice given in a timely manner. Case study 7.2 provides an example of this.

The timing of Kelly's interview is perfect! Her mentor has had four weeks to monitor her progress and there are still four weeks left for Kelly to work on any areas requiring improvement. Here the interview is truly a 'midpoint interview' as it is taking place exactly halfway through the placement. There has been time for her mentor Daniel to have supervised, facilitated, observed and assessed her learning. He will be able to draw on an adequate amount of data to review Kelly's progress to date. There is also, more importantly, adequate time left on the placement for Kelly to continue to progress towards achievement of the set learning outcomes and to work on areas identified as requiring attention and improvement. This is essential. Your student must have the time and the opportunity to show improvement between the midpoint and final interviews. If the time between midpoint and final interviews is too short, as in Gina's case, there will be few opportunities for the student to gain the knowledge and skills required and put these into practice. Without sufficient opportunity to try out new knowledge and skills in a variety of different settings, learning will not take place and your student will be unable to achieve the set outcomes. It is therefore crucial to schedule the midpoint interview to take place halfway through the placement.

Case study 7.2 Kelly's midpoint interview

It is Kelly's fourth week on Gladstone ward. Today she is meeting her mentor Daniel for her midpoint interview.

Daniel 'Hello Kelly. Thanks very much for coming in. You will be pleased to know we have about a good half hour to go through your midpoint interview and then I've got to go to a meeting, but I've handed the keys over to Sarah and she's going to hold the fort out on the ward. Is that your practice assessment book you've got there?' (Daniel takes the book and starts to flick through it). 'So how long have you been on this placement now?'

Kelly 'It's been three weeks. This is my fourth week now!'

Daniel 'Right, excellent! So you've got another four weeks to go then? Great!'

PLANNING FOR THE MIDPOINT INTERVIEW

The best way to ensure the midpoint interview is timely is to set the date for this during the initial interview. Setting the date well in advance provides opportunity for duty rosters to be organized to ensure that both you and your student's off-duty coincide. Advanced planning may also make it possible to choose a date when you anticipate the clinical workload will be less. For example if one day of the week is generally quieter than others as there is no theatre list, or there is a day when clinics finish earlier. Perhaps on your ward there is a patient rest period when no planned clinical interventions are carried out. All of these would be good times to choose. Taking time to consider clinical down times in advance will reduce the chance of the interview having to be postponed or interrupted. Of course, healthcare is unpredictable and there will always be occasions when despite advanced planning interviews will need to be rescheduled. The likelihood however of this happening is greatly reduced with a bit of forward planning. Remember also, that interview opportunities are increased the more shifts that you and your student are rostered together (Activity 7.2).

KEY POINT

Agree the date of the midpoint interview well in advanced, preferably during the initial interview. This will give plenty of time for off duties to be arranged and a target for your student to aim towards. Think about the clinical workload and try to identify periods when clinical activity is likely to be low.

Activity 7.2 Reasons for delayed midpoint interviews

Have a look again at the notes you took in Activity 7.1. If there were students who had a delayed midpoint interview then make some notes on why this happened. For example, were the mentor and student rostered together? Was the mentor on holidays? In doing this exercise you may be able to troubleshoot some of the common reasons that prevent timely midpoint interviews in your area.

LENGTH OF THE MIDPOINT INTERVIEW?

We have established that the timing of the midpoint interview is crucial, but how much time should you expect to allocate to it? To answer this question you might like to refer back to Case studies 7.1 and 7.2. In Case study 7.2, Daniel has set aside 30 minutes for his interview with Kelly whereas in Case study 7.1 Carol appears to have been caught 'on-the-hop' and so no actual time has been set aside. It is therefore highly unlikely that Gina's interview will last very long. Time is a precious resource within the healthcare environment so it is unlikely Carol, who is clearly unprepared for the encounter with Gina, will have time to spare. It is also obvious from the scenario that Carol and Gina have not planned the interview in advance so no time has been allocated to it.

Feedback sessions such as the midpoint interview are not effective if they are carried out hurriedly. If your student feels they pose an additional burden, in a busy clinical environment, they will be reluctant to approach you and their learning will suffer. We can see this in Gina's approach and response to Carol. She diminishes the importance of the interview, desperately trying to reassure Carol that 'It's nothing much', in other words it isn't going to take up much of Carol's precious time. 'You just need to sign to say how I'm getting on.' Gina obviously feels it is important to complete the assessment document. Perhaps she sees this as a way of keeping the university and her mentor happy. Her assessment book will have the required sections completed without making too many demands on her mentor's time. In effect two people lose out as a result of this scenario. Gina will receive no feedback on her performance and therefore lose any opportunity to improve. Carol loses out in that she has undermined her professional credibility and competence as a mentor. By not valuing the midpoint interview both the mentor and student lose out.

In Case study 7.2 Daniel is clearly expecting to do more than 'just . . . sign to say how Kelly is getting on'. Although 30 minutes may seem quite short, he has ensured the time will be devoted solely to Kelly as he has 'handed the keys over to Sarah [who is] going to hold the fort out on the ward'. He has taken steps to ensure that he will not be interrupted and is clearly sending a message to Kelly that he has the time to focus on her learning. Kelly will therefore feel valued and have a sense that her needs are considered to be important. It is also likely that this will make both Kelly and Daniel more relaxed and the interview more likely to be productive. Kelly will feel more able than Gina to discuss her learning needs with Daniel knowing that there are no other demands on his time. However, Daniel has also set a time limit. Kelly is fully aware at the very start of the interview how long it will last. Setting a definite time limit to the interview helps keep both you and your student focused. This reduces the chance of either of you going off on a tangent, keeping the focus strictly on reviewing progress towards achieving the outcomes.

You may decide towards the end of the allocated time that you need to meet again to discuss certain issues further but your student can act on the feedback received in the meantime.

> **KEY POINT**
>
> When arranging to carry out the midpoint interview make sure you choose a time when you will not be interrupted. Clearly define the length of the interview at the start and use the time productively.

WHERE SHOULD THE MIDPOINT INTERVIEW BE HELD?

When you are giving formal feedback to your student, it is crucial that you allocate sufficient time and space to the process to ensure that all aspects of the student's practice can be discussed without interruption. You also need to consider where the interview takes place. Ideally, the interview should take place in a quiet, private environment with an informal room layout to promote two-way discussion of the student's performance. The ward treatment room does not generally fit into this category and should be avoided, as constant interruptions will be stressful for both you and your student. Space, like time, is a precious commodity in healthcare environments; however, if planned in advanced it should be possible to ensure a private, quiet space is found.

RESPONSIBILITY FOR THE MIDPOINT INTERVIEW

Ultimately, it is the student's responsibility to ensure that all aspects of their practice assessment are completed correctly and on time. Many universities make the specific roles and responsibilities of the student and the mentor clear within the student practice assessment document, so that each party knows exactly where their respective responsibility lies. In adult education, the student is expected to take responsibility for their own learning and take the appropriate steps to ensure key stages in the learning process are achieved at the prescribed time. However, as we have seen in Chapter 2 the NMC sees it as the duty of every nurse and midwife to facilitate students to develop competence. This means that as a mentor you are responsible for ensuring students are given every opportunity to develop their level of competence. As we have seen above and in Chapter 6, in order to develop, students need regular constructive feedback, both informal and formal. Your student has a right to expect that you will point out any deficiencies in their performance and that you will provide guidance as to how they can improve – give constructive and timely feedback. You therefore have a professional responsibility to ensure that this happens.

Let's look at our two Case studies again. In Case study 7.1 Gina clearly demonstrates she is aware of her responsibility for ensuring the assessment process is followed. She has taken the initiative and asked to meet Carol. Carol does not appear to understand her role, asking Gina for guidance. She seems unaware of how far into her placement Gina is and seems unconcerned that the interview is almost three weeks late. Her comment to Gina that it 'doesn't matter, we can get something written down!' suggests that Carol lacks awareness of her responsibilities as a mentor. As a registered professional, Carol is accountable for the care given to patients/clients in her charge, whether this is care she personally delivers or care she delegates to others. She is therefore accountable for the care delivered by Gina. By failing to carry out a thorough midpoint interview and provide Gina with formal feedback on her progress, Carol may be putting her patients at risk. If Gina thinks she is progressing well she may attempt to carryout aspects of care in which she lacks sufficient competence and cause harm to a patient. If this were to happen, Carol as the registered professional supervising Gina's practice, would be answerable to both her employers and to the NMC. As a mentor, therefore, you have a professional and a moral responsibility to ensure the assessment process is fair and accurate.

KEY POINT

As a nurse you are accountable for the care you personally give to your patients but also for the care you delegate to others. It is therefore your responsibility to ensure that students under your supervision are aware of any weaknesses that may affect their competence in order to protect patients.

FEEDBACK AT THE MIDPOINT INTERVIEW

The midpoint interview is a formal stage of the continuous assessment process and although there are no hard and fast rules about what should and should not be said, there are a number of points that need to be addressed. Let's return to our two Case studies and see what happens next (Case studies 7.3 and 7.4).

Case study 7.3 Feedback at Kelly's midpoint interview

Daniel 'It's great to have this time to review the placement with you because we had the initial interview in the first week, didn't we? And we went through the different learning outcomes' (flicking through book). 'So just to recap, you're attempting 13 learning outcomes and there's two extra that you wanted to do yourself. So we will go through these in the next half hour. Just so you know I have talked to some of the other staff as well, the staff you have been working with because I know we haven't worked every shift, although we've been quite lucky doing quite a few shifts. But as I say I've talked to some of the other staff to get their feedback on how you've been doing and it's been really useful to get other people's view points. So I'll let you know what they said. OK?'
Kelly 'Yes. Thank you.'
Daniel 'So we need to look at the different learning outcomes. So if we start with the first one . . . . *Assess and plan patient's/client's care using a care pathway or an established framework* . . . How do you think you've been doing on that one?'

There are clearly very big differences in the way Carol and Daniel conduct the interview. Daniel sets out a clear agenda for the meeting and knows exactly what needs to be done. He appears to have prepared for the interview. Carol on the other hand doesn't seem very sure about what

Case study 7.4 Feedback at Gina's midpoint interview

Carol (Reading assessment book) 'So it's about student progress. Right! So, how are you progressing?'
Gina 'I'm really enjoying it. I'm having a great time. Everybody is really friendly and, you know, I can do stuff. I'm meeting people and . . .'
Carol (butting in) 'Good and you feel you are learning stuff and everything?'
Gina 'Yeh! Yeh'
Carol 'That's good! I know we haven't worked much together, well only a couple of times really, but I've not heard anything bad about you so that's good isn't it! All being well you should get through the placement without any problems. So everything's fine then!'

is involved. Daniel demonstrates he knows exactly what the purpose of the meeting is – to review Kelly's progress. He starts by revisiting the initial interview and learning plan. The initial interview is a good starting point for discussing progress. It is useful to remind students about the goals that were agreed and about how they felt and what they seemed anxious about. In the time between initial and midpoint interviews students can forget where they started and can focus too much on problems or worries that have arisen during the placement. As they gain competence and confidence they can forget what they didn't know and/or couldn't do so are unaware of the progress they have made. It is therefore important to point out exactly where progress has been made and remind your student about what they thought they didn't know or couldn't do at the start of the placement and the situations where they lacked confidence.

REFLECTION AT THE MIDPOINT INTERVIEW

In both Case studies, the mentor starts by asking the student to comment on their own progress. It is important to allow your student to assess their own learning, as self-assessment helps the student to take ownership of their learning and take control over the way they meet their learning needs. You need to remind your student of the ultimate goal of the placement and encourage them to articulate the progress they feel they have made so far. Skilful questioning can help learners identify any barriers to learning they are experiencing as well as enabling them to clarify any areas of misunderstanding that may have arisen. Daniel's approach is to refocus on the goals set in the initial interview, encouraging Kelly to reflect on how she is progressing towards achieving each one. By getting Kelly to describe her progress he is alerting her to her achievements.

CELEBRATING SUCCESS

It is vital that success and achievement are recognized at the midpoint interview as this helps motivate the student to strive for higher goals. Helping your student get a sense of his or her progress requires you to prompt them to recall what she or he could do or knew at the start of the placement. Reflecting back to where they started and comparing this with where they are now helps students to appreciate the range and complexity of learning to date. This is especially important for students who have made good progress in some areas but not in others. Helping them to appreciate just how much learning is involved (think of Kelly's

15 learning outcomes!) is one way of getting them to value their own efforts and appreciate why their progress may be uneven. It is important to remember as highlighted in Chapter 5 that each student you mentor will have a different style and capacity to learn. Some students will be practical hands-on learners who will acquire psychomotor skills easily. Others will be able to discuss rationale for care and excel in decision-making activities, whilst others will be good communicators, picking up the empathy and caring aspects of nursing naturally and easily. It is therefore important when celebrating your student's achievements to remind them that 'practice-based' learning requires the integration of knowledge and skills with praxis, that is, putting theory into action.

> **KEY POINT**
>
> The midpoint interview is a time to celebrate your student's successes, acknowledge competencies, and invite further thought and effort in areas that need improvement. The aim of this is to shift the student's focus from 'how good am I?' to 'how can I get better?' Discussing your student's progress towards achieving the learning outcomes agreed at the initial interview however involves more than just ticking boxes. You will need to encourage your student to reflect on how his/her performance compares to the benchmarks of good practice.

ENCOURAGING REFLECTION

Students should be encouraged to reflect on their own performance at the midpoint interview. In Case study 7.3 Daniel asks Kelly to reflect on how far she has come in achieving her first learning outcome by posing the question 'How do you think you've been doing on that one?' An alternative approach might be for Daniel to ask 'your outcome states that you should be able to assess and plan patient's/client's care using a care pathway or an established framework, but I wonder if you have thought about how well you have done.' Either way is fine and depends mainly on the language that you feel most comfortable and relaxed in using.

> **KEY POINT**
>
> It is important not only to help the student focus on achievements but also to establish what is good – what is above standard, what is OK – what is acceptable and where help is needed.

MEASURING PROGRESS AT THE MIDPOINT

It is important to compare the student's achievement at the midpoint interview with what they were expected to achieve. If goals or targets have not been met, you will need to explore the reasons for this. You will also need to consider whether the goals set were realistic given the time and opportunities available to the student. It is also important to discuss any specific problems the student may have encountered, for example accessing the necessary patient care experiences.

It is also crucial that you clearly articulate to the student any problem areas that need addressing. As highlighted in Chapter 6 what you think you have said is not always what the student hears. Use clear language avoiding euphemisms and check your student has understood. However, try to use as non-evaluative language as possible, for example 'Have you thought about asking the patient. . .?' rather than 'Your questioning of the patient was totally inadequate.' When highlighting weaknesses avoid generalizations. Give the student specific examples: 'remember last Tuesday when we were completing the admission interview with Mr Sing I had to remind you to ask him about . . . and again on Friday with Mr Short' rather than 'there have been lots of times when we have been working together when I have had to remind you to ask . . ..' This will help the student view the comments in context and make it clearer what the weaknesses are. Using examples to emphasize your points also helps to keep the interview constructive, objective and based in fact rather than straying into your personal opinion.

KEY POINT

Use clear language and specific examples to help the student recognize strengths and weaknesses.

FEEDBACK FROM OTHER HEALTH PROFESSIONALS

It is unlikely that prior to the interview your student will have worked exclusively with you and therefore you will need to obtain feedback from colleagues. Second- or third-hand feedback, for example, 'staff nurse Jones says that you are. . .' is never as persuasive as your own personal observations, as the student may be less likely to accept the criticism, especially if the originator of the feedback has not discussed the problem or issue with the student in person. Written comments or testimonies like the example shown in Box 7.1 may be a more powerful way of utilizing feedback from other healthcare professionals.

Box 7.1 Witness testimony for student nurse Kelly Smith

During an afternoon shift Mary was assisting in the care of a patient in HDU. The patient was on wall CPAP and was finding it difficult to cope with the mask and kept taking it off. Unfortunately, this caused his saturations to drop markedly so we were particularly keen that he keep his mask on for as long as possible to avoid intubation. Mary was given the task of reassuring the patient and persuading him to keep his mask on. She carried out this task exceptionally well. Talking to the patient about his family, what was in the paper that morning and how well he was progressing. She was also able to empathize with the patient, telling him that she understood how uncomfortable the mask was, and having first checked with the doctor and myself that it was OK, removed the mask for short periods to moisten the patient's lips and mouth.

Mary had cared for the patient the previous day and had obviously developed a good relationship with him. She had found out all the names of his family and had obviously talked to some of them the previous day, as she seemed to know a great deal about each of them. This enabled her to really communicate with the patient. He obviously found this reassuring and he seemed to trust her.

Mary also displayed real compassion in caring for this patient. She was exceptionally gentle with him, spoke softly and used gentle persuasion to get his co-operation. Without Mary's help that day I don't think we would have avoided reintubation.

DOCUMENTING AT THE MIDPOINT INTERVIEW

As the midpoint interview is a formal stage of the assessment process there needs to be a written record that it has taken place. At the end of the interview therefore, you will need to write a summary of the discussion. Most practice assessment documents include a section where both the mentor and student record their comments. Refer back to Chapter 4 for more detail about this. Without a written record of the event there is no evidence to support what has been discussed and the agreed actions to be taken. As discussed in Chapter 2 you are accountable and responsible to the NMC for decisions you make regarding a student's fitness to practice. This means that your written record must be an accurate summary of what has taken place. In the document *Standards to Support Learning and Assessment in Practice* (NMC, 2008) the NMC highlight the importance of written records regarding student assessment. Within these standards the NMC highlight that mentors must maintain an audit trail to support their decision. In addition, where a critical decision on progress is to be made the mentor should ensure that regular feedback is given to the student and that records are kept of guidance given. The midpoint interview would be an example of such a time.

What you write therefore needs to be an accurate reflection of the interview. You need to be clear and concise in the language you use. As with verbal feedback, avoid ambiguities and euphemisms. Stipulate exactly what the student's achievements to date have been, providing examples of good practice. You must also clearly identify the areas where improvement or further practice is required, again providing examples. A comprehensive account of the midpoint interview will help you reach your final summative judgement and record the student's learning journey. Once again there are Case studies that highlight the differences in midpoint interview documentation (Case studies 7.5 and 7.6).

Case study 7.5 Summary of Kelly's midpoint interview

Student comments

I feel I am progressing and have achieved some of my learning outcomes (3a,b,c; 4a,d,e,f; 5a–f). I agree I still need to improve in aspects of drug administration – knowledge of how drugs work and injection technique. I still find it difficult to explain why I am doing things but I am motivated and willing to learn. I also find it difficult sometimes to get my work completed on time and get flustered when there are lots of things happening or need to be done. I think I will get more organized with more experience.

Mentor's comments

Kelly is improving slowly. She is motivated and trying well. She is aware now of emergency procedures and where we keep equipment on the ward. Her nursing care is generally very good and she was praised a few times by patients. She has made progress towards achieving several of her outcomes and has achieved competence in 12. Her weak area is general knowledge of medication and illnesses and she is not aware of the rationale behind basic things like why a patient is on a fluid chart. She is improving with her time management but still needs reminding to organise her work so she finishes it all on time. We have agreed action plans to address these areas.

Signature of Student: *Kelly Jones* Date: 26/10/09
Signature of Mentor: *Daniel Wright* Date: 26/10/09

Case study 7.6 *Summary of Gina's midpoint interview*

Student comments

I am progressing and achieving some of my learning and am working hard to achieve knowledge and expertise to care safely for patients. My mentor has stressed to me the importance of continuing to work hard.

Practice assessor's comments

Gina has settled into the ward well and is making good progress with her learning outcomes. Although I have not had much opportunity to work with her my colleagues have found her to be a willing worker and learner.

Signature of Student: Gina Suleman Date: 26/10/09

Signature of Mentor: Carol Mills Date: 26/10/09

The comments provided by Daniel give a clear indication of the progress made by Kelly, celebrating her achievements. He also identifies clearly Kelly's areas of weakness. In contrast, Carol's comments do not tell us what Gina has or has not achieved. There is nothing in this account that can be used to measure Gina's progress over the remaining weeks. We do not know what outcomes have been achieved and which are outstanding. There is nothing in this account to provide guidance to Gina of how to progress further.

KEY POINT

When writing a summary of the midpoint interview identify the student's strengths and weaknesses. Clearly state what learning outcomes have been achieved and be specific about the areas of weakness. Provide sufficient detail so that other professionals will be able to facilitate the student's learning.

ACTION PLANNING

The final stage of the midpoint interview is the completion of an action plan. Action planning is a process that helps the student focus and decide what steps need to be taken to achieve their goals. An effective action plan should give the student a concrete timetable and a set of clearly defined steps to help them reach their objectives. Action planning involves:

- identifying specific objectives
- setting objectives which are SMART
- identifying the steps needed to achieve objectives
- identifying appropriate resources and strategies.

Learning objectives are statements of intent, that is, what the student will achieve. Setting specific objectives provides direction for learning and act as the criteria against which progress can be measured. To be effective they need to be *s*pecific, *m*easurable, *a*chievable, *r*elevant, and *t*ime bound (SMART). We first looked at SMART learning outcomes in Chapter 4 in terms of the learning outcomes that come pre-determined within the student's practice assessment document by the university.

However, at the midpoint interview there will be an opportunity to set new learning goals for the placement, and these too must be SMART. Box 7.2 presents the SMART criteria that will be applicable in this instance. While very similar to the SMART criteria outlined in Chapter 4, there are some minor differences.

Box 7.2 SMART outcomes for specific objectives

- *Specific*; accurately state what the student is expected to achieve in terms of knowledge and skills, which might be intellectual or practical skills, and attitudes and values. Are presented in terms of what the student will (not should) know or be able to do.
- *Measurable*; are observable and assessable, i.e. clearly state the behaviour the student will demonstrate to show they have achieved the outcome. When setting learning objectives you need to incorporate action verbs: e.g. compile, create, plan, revise, analyse, design, select, utilize, apply, demonstrate, prepare, use, compute, discuss, explain, predict, assess, compare, rate, critique.

Verbs that are unclear and subject to different interpretations in terms of what action they are specifying should not be used in a learning objective. Such verbs call for covert behaviour, which cannot be observed or measured: e.g. know, become aware of, appreciate, learn, understand, become familiar with.

- *Achievable*: are within the student's range of abilities.
- *Relevant*: i.e. relate to the weaknesses highlighted in the formative assessment.
- *Time scaled*: have clear target dates set for achievement.

Box 7.3 Developing an action plan

Date	Area of concern	Goal/outcome	Learning opportunities/ resources	Review date
6/10/09	Knowledge of medication	I will be able to explain to my mentor how the following drugs work: Frusemide; digoxin; metformin; nifedipine; flucloxacillin, aspirin	When working with Daniel we will do drug rounds together. I will look up the drugs in the BNF. I will read up on the drugs in the ward book *Basic Pharmacology for Nurses.* Daniel will test me on what I know each time we work together.	26/10/09

Name of Mentor: Daniel Wright Signature: Daniel Wright
Name of student: Kelly Jones Signature: Kelly Jones

The resources, learning opportunities and experiences the student will need to access to achieve the set objective must also be identified. This will enable the student to work independently as well as focus time spent working alongside you. An example of Kelly's action plan is represented in Box 7.3.

SEEKING HELP AT THE MIDPOINT INTERVIEW

A separate action plan should be completed for each area of weakness identified in the interview. Clear target dates should be set so that progress can be monitored and ongoing problems can be identified before the end of the placement. When a student is failing to meet the set targets you must inform the university link lecturer. The link lecturer may be able to provide extra help and guidance to the student and may also arrange for an additional period of practice. Remember not all students will learn at the same speed. Some students will need a longer time to practise skills and apply theory to practice than others. If you can help them identify weaknesses early and provide the necessary support and guidance through the provision of clear action plans their learning journey will be made much easier.

KEY POINT

If you would like a link lecturer to be present during a midpoint interview then ask them in good time and fix a date so they can diary it in. Don't forget to tell the student, so they are also prepared to see the link lecturer.

MAKING THE MOST OF THE MIDPOINT INTERVIEW

The midpoint interview is an important stage in the continuous assessment process. It is a formal formative stage and should provide the student with a clear sense of their achievements and their ongoing learning needs. It should be carried out halfway through the student's placement. This ensures you have had sufficient opportunity to observe the student in practice to be able to assess their progress towards achieving the final learning outcomes. It also ensures the student has sufficient time for further practice on any areas of weakness.

You will need to provide a concise summary of your discussions with the student. This will allow you and the student to measure progress between the midpoint and final summative assessment stages. You will also need to agree action plans for any weaknesses identified so that there is a clear plan of learning to assist the student to achieve the placement outcomes. Your written record of the interview and subsequent action plans can then be used to measure your student's progress in the time remaining.

Like all aspects of the mentoring process, confidence is vital. Rather than avoiding a midpoint interview, try to view it as an invaluable tool to assess not only your student's progress, but your performance as a mentor during the placement. If there are any aspects of your role as a mentor that require improvement, then the midpoint interview is an ideal time to identify where and how to improve. Following the midpoint interview both you and your student can move together into the second half of the placement with renewed enthusiasm and respect for each other's contribution to the learning experience.

TOP TIPS

- Plan for the midpoint interview. If possible agree a specific date at the initial interview.
- Allocate a specific time and room for the midpoint interview. This will indicate to the student that their progress is important to you.
- Seek help for action planning if you need help with this skill.
- Use the feedback sandwich for written and verbal feedback. Your student needs a clear indication of where and how to improve, but they will also benefit from a good helping of praise.

CHAPTER 8

SUPPORTING THE FAILING STUDENT

Chapter Aims

The purpose of this chapter is to develop skills for supporting a student who is failing to achieve their learning outcomes at important stages during the practice placement. After reading this chapter you will be able to:

- Identify the early warning signs of failing students.
- Understand the importance of accessing help and support for failing students early in the placement.
- Develop action plans to support the failing student.

WHAT DO WE MEAN BY FAILING?

The word fail is a highly emotive word. No one likes to be told they have failed. In reality very few students actually fail their practice assessment. The correct term used by universities to describe a student who has not met the required standard of competence for one or more learning outcomes in their practice assessment at their first attempt is *referred*. A student is only deemed to have failed when it is their final attempt at an assessment. The main focus of this chapter is on students who are failing to achieve the required standard of competence and the steps you can take to turn this around.

MENTORING CHALLENGES – THE FAILING STUDENT

Being the mentor of a student who is failing to achieve the required standard is one of the biggest challenges you will face. The nature of the event means that it is never a pleasant experience and can be equally traumatic for mentor and student alike. In fact, a failing student is one of the more common reasons for mentors wishing to disengage from mentoring students. Without adequate preparation, supporting a student who is failing to achieve the required standard through their placement can give rise to a whole series of problems for you, the student, future mentors and the university.

affiliated university, the competencies you are assessing will have been based upon the proficiencies set by the NMC and have been interpreted into separate learning outcomes or competencies which the student has to achieve. This means that as a mentor you are professionally accountable and responsible for the assessment decision that you make to the NMC.

As the mentor of a student on placement you are required to fulfil two roles, to facilitate learning experiences related to the learning outcomes and to assess the student's competence related to those outcomes. Your decision regarding their competence will be related to three themes:

- knowledge
- skill
- attitude.

So, just as you are facilitating learning experiences that relate to these three attributes, you will be determining competence that directly relates to knowledge, skill and attitude.

KEY POINT

Make a point of reading the NMC *Standards for Pre-registration Nursing Education* (available from www.nmc-uk.org) for yourself and discuss these with your colleagues so you are clear regarding the standards of competence to expect from students.

WHY IS MY STUDENT FAILING?

When faced with a failing student situation on a placement, many mentors may conclude that the placement has 'gone wrong'. It stems from a misguided disbelief that if you are a good mentor your students always pass; only poor mentors have students that fail. This is not true at all. While poor mentorship can contribute to a student's poor performance, even the best mentors will be faced at some point with a student who is unable to meet the required level of competence. There is no evidence that a student's ability or success is directly proportional to the skill of a mentor. So when you are faced with a failing student your reaction should never be 'why me?' as this would suggest that you have some sort of superhuman ability to attract only students who will succeed every time. Rather you should focus on the influence you have as a mentor to help the student achieve the best level of competence they can.

FAILING DURING THE PLACEMENT

There are two main ways that students 'fail' during a practice placement. Some students may initially be judged to be failing to achieve the required standard of competence during the early part of their placement, but may improve their performance and the end result may be a pass. Other students may fail to reach the required level of competence during their placement and despite appropriate interventions fail to improve; with the end result a failure to achieve one or more learning outcomes. Whichever is the case, failing to meet the required level of competence at any stage during a placement means that you have a failing student situation. For a student to be considered to be failing there must be a deficit in their knowledge, skills or attitudes or a combination of all three.

ALARM BELLS START RINGING

If you do have concerns regarding your student's knowledge, skill or attitude related to any learning outcome during a placement then alarm bells should start ringing. This will be the first warning sign that there may be a potential problem and you should never ignore this. Hoping that a problem will just go away if you don't think about it or given more time will never be the solution and you will only make matters worse for your student and yourself if you take this approach. You must take action as soon as you realize there may be a problem with competence.

If you have not conducted a timely or thorough initial interview then it may take some time before the alarm bells really start ringing. Even when you do identify concerns, without a well documented initial interview it will be more difficult to nail down the exact aspect of competence that you are concerned about. If you are unsure of, or confused about, the student's learning outcomes valuable time will be lost in trying to identify the actual problem. Case study 8.2 provides an example of how things can go wrong.

If a student is falling short of the required level of competence then they need help. More importantly, it is part of your professional role as a mentor to provide this help. If you do not take steps to identify the problem and assist the failing student then both of you are failing in this situation.

WHAT IS THE PROBLEM?

The first step you must take when identifying a failing student is to ascertain exactly what the concern is. There must be evidence related to your concern not just a hunch or a feeling. In Case study 8.2, Jane had

Case study 8.2 *A mentor's experience of identifying a student that needs support*

Jane is mentoring Peter, a final year child branch student. Jane works in a children's day treatment centre where there is a high turnover of children every day and staff are constantly busy. Jane is concerned about Peter's communication skills with the parents of the children they are treating. He lacks confidence when speaking to the parents and avoids eye contact with them. Some parents have commented on his lack of engagement with them. Jane did not get a chance to look at Peter's learning outcomes during the initial interview and it is the third week of Peter's placement before she looks at the assessment book during the midpoint interview. To her horror she realizes that there is a specific learning outcome that requires her to assess Peter's confidence in communicating with children and parents. Jane realizes that Peter is currently failing in this area, but the placement is now halfway over and valuable time has been lost. Jane finds herself having to tell Peter that he is failing a learning outcome with very little time left to improve. She feels guilty and angry that her manager has made her mentor students when the unit is so busy.

concerns related to Peter's communication. This needed to be evidenced by examples where his communication had been unsatisfactory. In this case it was verbal communication and evidence could be given related to specific examples of his poor communication with relatives as well as the feedback Jane had received from some of them.

While a one-off event may be a very early warning of a problem with competence, it is rarely a good idea to base your decision on just one example. If your student is weak in an aspect of competence then it is preferable that there are several examples of this to evidence your concerns. However, if the area in which a student is weak could lead to harm then you clearly should not wait for the student to continue in this way.

You must be very clear in your own mind what it is that you are concerned about and what aspect of competence this relates to before addressing the issue with your student. This does not mean that you should wait for weeks before discussing your concerns, rather, you should move very quickly to decide if there really is a problem and if so, the exact nature of your concerns. Try to be very clear about whether you are concerned with a student's knowledge, skill or their attitude, and have examples of how these concerns have been demonstrated in practice. Once again, if you have completed a thorough initial interview you should have a very clear benchmark on which to base your decision.

> **KEY POINT**
>
> If you do have concerns regarding a student's competence then make a quick note of the event, time and date so you can refer to this accurately if needed.

AM I BEING TOO HARSH?

It is poor practice to rely solely on your own opinion when deciding upon a student's competence. As a mentor you should make every effort to consult with your colleagues to gain their judgements of your student's ability, particularly if you believe there may be a problem. While one person's opinion could be subjective, a number of different opinions will dramatically increase the objectivity of an assessment decision. This is referred to as inter-assessor reliability. Ask your colleagues if they have noticed any particular issues or have examples of practice that support your concerns. If no one else has noticed a problem then it may be that you are expecting a higher standard than is required for the student at their particular stage on the programme and you may need to adjust your own expectations. Alternatively, you may like to ask your fellow mentors to undertake their own assessment of the student in the areas you are concerned about. If others are equally concerned regarding a student's competence then this is the time to discuss your concerns with your student.

> **KEY POINT**
>
> Discuss with your colleagues the attributes of competence that will be expected for the range of learning outcomes commonly assessed in your area. In this way all mentors in the placement will have a benchmark by which to make their judgements.

DISCUSSING COMPETENCE WITH STUDENTS

Once you have determined that there is a particular area in which your student is failing to reach the expected level of competence in then you must address this as soon as possible with them. You must be very clear regarding what your concerns are, why you are concerned and provide them with evidence of your concerns. This should be based on very identifiable situations or events that have taken place during the placement that support your concerns related to their knowledge, skill or attitude. It is never easy to hear that you are falling short of a standard, so be gentle and considerate in your approach when discussing these problems with a student. However, above all be honest. If there is a problem then your student must be very clear about what it is, as they will need to know exactly what is wrong before they can take steps to improve. Discussing with a student your concerns regarding their level of competence and what can be done may not always get the reaction you expect (see Case study 8.3).

Case study 8.3 *A student speaks of her experience of feedback*

'The best placement I ever had was actually one that I failed in the end. My mentor was just so up front and honest and I'm really grateful to her for that. I was so nervous and shy in my first year, and had a lot of trouble adjusting to speaking in public. I would go into handover to talk about my patients and just freeze, I'd try to talk but nothing would happen. She was just so kind in trying to help. We tried everything, I'd do a practice handover with her, or write out what I was going to say, but it just got worse. I was a wreck. In the end she suggested that the best option was to accept that I wouldn't achieve that outcome on this placement and plan for how I could achieve confidence slowly and pass at a second attempt. Just having the pressure off and knowing I had more time made all the difference. I was so pleased that I failed because I got more time on my second attempt and didn't have the pressure of going into second year with this hanging over my head.'

In Chapter 6 we discussed feedback in depth, and you should refer to the advice provided in that chapter when discussing problems with competence with your student. You will need to be quite skilled yourself in delivering accurate feedback as what you say and the way you say it will make all the difference. As a general rule, everything you say at this stage should be directly related to the learning outcomes the student is attempting, and be supported by as many specific examples as necessary.

WHAT IF MY STUDENT DENIES THERE IS A PROBLEM?

One of the more difficult aspects of mentoring a failing student occurs when your student denies that there is a problem with their competence. In this situation there are only two possible explanations, and only one of you can be right. Either:

1. You have got it wrong – there may be no problem with the student's competence

or

2. You have got it right and there is a problem with their competence.

HAVE YOU GOT IT WRONG?

If a student denies that there is a problem with their competence then it is quite likely that you may begin to doubt your own assessment skills. You may ask yourself if you have made the right decision. Perhaps you might begin to doubt your own mind. Most mentors will have the same feelings when faced with an outright denial from a student. Of course, there is always the chance that you may have made an incorrect decision. If you are basing your assessment of competence on something other than a learning outcome, or you have no supporting evidence of why you are concerned then you could well be in the wrong and a student has every right to challenge this. You must therefore be very sure of your concerns and facts before discussing failings of competence with a student, which means preparing before meeting with the student so you have all the evidence at hand. Remember that the chances of you reaching an incorrect conclusion will be reduced if you have sought the opinion of others and are not just relying on your own assessment abilities.

STUDENTS IN DENIAL

The other explanation of course is that you have made the correct assessment, but your student may deny that there is a problem with their competence. This is a very difficult situation for a mentor; however it is quite common for a student to deny problems with their own competence. Your student is not setting out to make your role difficult, it's just fact that some students will genuinely believe they have no problems and may have little insight into what you are raising as a problem. It takes considerable reflective ability to recognize problems in ourselves, and some students may find it difficult to see where they are failing. In other words they can't know what they don't know. This can be really challenging for you as a mentor but it is important that you stick to your judgement; you are the expert when it comes to the real world of practice, not the student (see Case study 8.4).

Case study 8.4 A mentor speaks about a failing student

'A few years ago I had to fail a student and it was very difficult at the time because he just refused to accept there were any problems. He had a lot of trouble reading prescription charts and if I hadn't been supervising him on drug rounds he would have overdosed many patients. I would explain this to him but he would just deny it. Other mentors had the same experience so I knew it wasn't me. It was very difficult to give him any help because he just refused to admit there was a problem. The university lecturer was very supportive and when I did fail him in the end she supported me in making the right decision. He wasn't happy but my conscience was clear.'

GIVING FEEDBACK TO FAILING STUDENTS

The first step is to ask the student how they believe they are doing. If you are lucky they may identify concern about the same areas as you which will make it easier to then discuss how this will be managed. Unfortunately, it is more likely they will say all is well and you then have to tell them about your concerns.

Even though your feedback may be unpopular, your student will be relying on you as their mentor, having identified their deficiencies, to now explore with them how they can be addressed. Giving feedback and then agreeing actions is part of your professional role as a mentor. If your student does not believe that there is a problem then they will naturally deny it exists. This is where the evidence of your concerns will be vital. You will need to very calmly and gently provide your student with evidence that demonstrates their lack of competence in order for them to understand that there is a problem at all. Without evidence your discussion can become a case of your word against theirs and you will end up in a very uncomfortable stalemate.

Your evidence should be conclusive without being overwhelming. Try to have a couple of key examples to hand that support why you have reason to be concerned. Ideally, this should include some instances where you were involved in an activity together so you can refer to specific events within the experience. You should also ensure that your student is aware that other mentors/staff are equally concerned and that this is not just your opinion. If you have informed the student at the initial interview that their assessment will be based on evidence from a wide variety of sources this information should be reassuring rather than provoke conflict.

BE OBJECTIVE

It is vitally important at this stage that you keep your personal opinion out of the concerns you raise. While it is true that you are the assessor, you should make it very clear that you are basing your assessment on NMC standards, and not your own personal agenda and that your feedback is about their competence and not about them as a person. This is the time more than ever to be as objective as possible and keep the subjective elements to a minimum. Where possible reinforce that the problem or problems have been noted by a range of staff rather than just you. Once faced with specific and clear examples of your particular concerns most students will agree to some extent that there is a problem to be resolved and will want to work with you to resolve the problem.

EARLY FAILURE DOES NOT MEAN END FAILURE

If you do notice that a student is struggling to meet the required standard of competence during their placement then it is very important that you distinguish between failing during the placement and failing at the end of the placement. Failing during the placement means that the required standard is not currently being reached, however, a final decision has not been made and there is time to improve.

Failing the placement can only happen at the end of the placement and is the result of failure to reach the required standard of competence in one or more learning outcomes by the end of the placement. This is another reason to raise your concerns early with a student. An early warning of potential failure provides maximum opportunity to improve and decreases the possibility of end failure. Late warning of failure limits opportunities to improve and actually promotes failure. Where possible, try to raise concerns as soon as you notice problems, within days of first identifying a problem if possible. Do not make the mistake of waiting weeks to raise problems with a student, or waiting for the midpoint interview so that you can raise your concerns. All you will be doing in this instance is denying your student the time which they need to improve.

KEY POINT

Alert your student as soon as possible if you have any concerns regarding their performance. This will give the student time to take appropriate actions to improve.

HELPING FAILING STUDENTS

While raising concerns with a student regarding their competence is an important part of your mentoring role, your responsibility does not end there. Your role also entails offering help and support to enable the student to improve on the problem you have identified. In fact you should not raise any concerns regarding competence with a student unless you are also prepared to offer a solution. You should therefore ensure that you have the time and resources to provide feedback and the necessary ongoing support.

The act of offering help and support when identifying problems with students also lessens the emotional impact of the feedback they receive. If a student is given clear feedback from you that you can back up with a clear offer of support then they will be far more willing to respect your assessment. By exploring how you can help the student they will be far more willing to accept that there is a problem that needs resolving.

ACTION PLANS

The best support that you can offer a student will involve the development of a clear plan of action. The action plan should clearly indicate the exact nature of the problem you have identified and include clear steps that will be provided to support the student. They should be involved in the development of the action plan as much as possible as they need to take ownership of the problem and the actions agreed. The focus should not be on the problem, rather on what they can do about it with your support. Ideally, an action plan should cover the following elements (Table 8.1):

1. The date the action plan is developed
2. The exact nature of the problem, including the learning outcome the problem is related to

Date	Area of concern	Objectives for competence	Plan of support	Review date

Table 8.1 An example of an action plan

Date	Area of concern	Objectives for competence	Plan of support	Review date
26/08/ 2010	Jenny is very nervous during ward handover and has not been able to report clear patient progress to members of the team. As a result she is not achieving learning outcome 7.	Jenny will need to develop confidence in handing over patient care which is accurate and of sufficient detail during ward meetings in order to achieve learning outcome 7.	1. Jenny will be given the opportunity to write out her notes to read out prior to the handover meeting. 2. Jenny will practice her handover with her mentor prior to handover to the team. 3. Jenny will be encouraged to handover at least three patients she has been caring for by the end of week 6.	08/09/ 2010

3. What needs to be to achieved to demonstrate competence
4. What help will be available to the student to improve their competence
5. A date to review the action plan.

The important features of an action plan are that problems are clearly identified, that there is a clear indication of what needs to be improved on and how this can be achieved with examples of the support that will be offered. However, the most important element is agreeing what the student will need to demonstrate in order to show that they have achieved the required standard of competence. If you are unclear as to what they need to do how can you know if they have achieved it? The action plan will provide an additional benchmark that can be referred to as evidence of continued development and demonstrates evidence that you are following the assessment process. A documented action plan provides evidence that you are fulfilling your professional accountability and responsibility as a mentor, by facilitating learning opportunities and undertaking a fair and accurate assessment.

GETTING HELP FOR FAILING STUDENTS

If your student is failing to meet the required standard of competence in any learning outcomes it is appropriate to seek additional help. This is no time to go it alone and hope you can manage to get it right. Requesting help at this stage will ensure you make the best possible decisions for your student.

SUPPORT FROM COLLEAGUES

The most obvious and immediate support available to you will be your own colleagues. There may be a number of people available to help you including:
- senior mentors
- unit managers
- practice educators
- placement facilitators.

Who you turn to for support is essentially down to you and will probably be dictated by local policies or your professional relationships. The main point is that you do seek help early in the assessment process. A failing student will increase your workload as you will need to factor in additional time to spend with them action planning, providing support and delivering feedback. This is the time to ensure your colleagues rally around you and share the load where practical.

UNIVERSITY SUPPORT

You must also inform the university when a student is failing to reach the required standard of competence in one or more learning outcomes. The university should be made aware as soon as a problem is identified so that support measures can be put in place for both you and the student. It is a common myth that the university only needs to be informed that a student has failed at the end of a placement. This is not correct. The NMC makes it very clear that as a mentor you are entitled to a network of support and this should be available to you throughout the placement and not just at the end. If a student is failing to reach the required standard then you will need access to this support. The people available to help you may be any or all of the following:

- link lecturers
- lecturer practitioners
- practice educators
- programme leaders
- personal tutors.

Most universities have a dedicated practice team so there will be people available who can be called upon to support mentors of failing students, and also support the students themselves. Do not be embarrassed to access this support and use the expertise and help available.

DON'T FORGET TO DOCUMENT

Throughout the whole of the student placement there should be clear and accurate records maintained in the student's assessment documentation of their progress or lack of it. There will be formal records at the initial, midpoint and end interview stage and there are chapters in this book dedicated to these stages of the student placement. However, additional records should also be maintained for significant events throughout a student's placement. You should therefore aim to keep very clear records of any actions you take related to a failing student. While action plans may form part of this documentation you may like to consider keeping additional records. This type of documentation can be used to keep a clear record of student progress and also to provide evidence of the help and support you have provided a failing student. The types of records you may like to consider include the following:

- specific learning objectives that are of concern
- reasons and evidence of concern
- summary of feedback and discussions with student
- help provided, dates, people involved, etc.
- documented action plans.

The NMC advises that a clear audit trail is kept of assessment decisions but does not expect these to be kept separately but recorded within the student's assessment document, using additional pages where necessary.

At all stages in the placement you must be up front and honest with your student. As soon as you recognize problems during the placement you must ensure that they know exactly where they stand and the help and support you are offering. Document all these offers of support. Make sure you base your documentation on fact, and ensure the student feels a part of the action plan for success. Consistent and honest feedback will be essential. If improvement is being made then make sure the student is aware of this and document what progress is being made. If improvement in competence is not being made then also ensure the student is kept informed and continue to document your concerns. The more information the student receives regarding their progress the better, and there should be records to support all this.

MAKING THE FINAL ASSESSMENT DECISION

The support you provide a failing student during a placement is vital for three reasons.
1. A failing student can improve if offered help and support.
2. Due process can be shown so ensuring the assessment process is valid.
3. The help and support you provide acts as evidence that you have fulfilled you responsibility and accountability as a mentor.

Unfortunately, it is often the case that despite all support and advice, some students will not reach the required standard of competence in all areas and therefore cannot be signed-off as having achieved all their learning outcomes. Your final assessment decision will therefore be to record 'not achieved' or an unsatisfactory grade by the relevant outcomes. You must not take this personally. Providing help and support no matter how good it is or how dedicated you have been will not always lead to success. Unfortunately, some students will be unable to respond sufficiently within the time frame given. What is important is that the support and help you provide demonstrates that you have provided the student with every opportunity to improve.

KEY POINT

If it is a student's first attempt, rather than tell them that they have failed their assessment, tell them that you will have to refer them on certain learning outcomes. This is in keeping with university terminology and the word *refer* is less emotive than *fail*.

FEELING GUILTY

If your student does not achieve the required standard of competence with regards to some of their learning outcomes then your professional role requires that you identify that on those specific outcomes. Most mentors will find this a very unpleasant and harrowing event. It is common for mentors to feel quite guilty and remorseful, as they feel responsible for the impact this will have on the student's future.

In these circumstances it is often the case that mentors fail to fail. Even though they are fully aware that the student is not competent, they will justify their decision not to fail in a desperate attempt to not face the reality of the situation. The fact is that most mentors who fail to fail do so because of what they perceive will be the negative consequences of their decision to fail on the student or how they will be perceived by the student. They may wish to dis-associate themselves from these perceived negative consequences by avoiding the decision, or deferring the decision to someone else. This type of 'passing the buck' attitude will only serve to create significant problems for the student and future mentors but is also a failure by the mentor to take accountability for their decisions. Undertake Activity 8.1 to explore your own experience of failing students.

Activity 8.1 Personal reflection on failing students

Mentors 'fail to fail' for a number of different reasons. Take some time now to reflect on your own personal experience of mentoring, perhaps a time or situation where you or others have failed to fail. Consider:
1. How did this situation arise?
2. What was the main reason that you or others failed to fail a student who was not competent?
You may find that it helps to write down the key issues that you feel impacted on the situation.

FAILING TO FAIL

Failure to fail often happens when mentors feel a lack of support for or confidence in their mentoring role. It can also happen when mentors have not fulfilled their mentoring role during a placement (e.g. lack of feedback, no or delayed midpoint interview) and wish to avoid conflict with their student at the final assessment. Some of the more common reasons include:

- Failure to establish the expected standard of competence for each learning outcome. Mentors may fail to fail if they are unsure of what standard of competence should be expected by the student. Under these circumstances mentors pass students who have 'worked hard' or 'shown enthusiasm' as they are confused themselves regarding the proficiencies they should be assessing.
- Failure to consistently assess a student's competence throughout the placement. Mentors may fail to fail simply because they did not witness the student's performance and base their final assessment on a limited number of interactions. This situation can easily arise if the mentor and student are not rostered together.
- Failure to highlight concerns with competence in the placement. Mentors may fail to fail if they do not raise their concerns regarding student's competence throughout the placement. This situation can easily arise when mentors hope that the student will improve without the need to raise concerns and inform the university. If the student has not been informed of concerns throughout the placement there is a high likelihood of conflict at the end. Mentors may then fail to fail in order to avoid potential conflict.
- Failure to recognize professional accountability and responsibility. Mentors may fail to fail if they feel that they are not required to make this decision. They may feel that it is the responsibility of more senior mentors or the university's responsibility to fail a student on their assessments.

The key point here is in that all the above examples of failure to fail the person who has failed is the mentor. If you fail to fail then you have failed in your professional role. Whether it is failure to work consistently with a student, or failure to assess outcomes accurately, the failure is yours. Remember you are accountable and responsible to the NMC for your assessment decisions.

FAILING WITH KINDNESS

The kindest thing that you can do for a failing student once all support has been put in place and is still unable to achieve the required standard is to fail them. The worst thing you could possibly do is pass a student who has not met a competent standard. To pass an incompetent student denies them access to the help and support they need. An incorrect assessment does not mean that the student is competent; rather, they and others will be under the impression that no more help or support is required in this area. The student will be left struggling with no plan or process for improving their area of weaknesses.

By failing a student you are making a professional decision and demonstrating you understand your own accountability and responsibility. You will have highlighted that there is a particular problem that requires support for the student to be put in place with a focused plan to guide improvement. You will have flagged up a student that needs help and provided a way for them to get help. Failing a student brings in the cavalry. If you highlight competency problems early in a student's placement then you are giving them every chance to improve. If the improvement is not sufficient during the placement then failing them at the final assessment means that the student can continue to be supported with regards to the issues of concern raised once the placement has finished. Nothing you say or do should come as a surprise to the student, especially if you have raised your concerns regarding performance early in the placement and provided consistent and honest feedback.

ONGOING ACHIEVEMENT RECORD

The reasons as to why a student has failed to reach a competent standard must also be documented in their ongoing achievement record. This is not only your summary of the events that took place on the placement; it is also your opportunity to inform the next mentor regarding support the student requires. The more detailed you can be about specific concerns you have and the support the student will require, the more help the next mentor can provide.

> **KEY POINT**
>
> When you write the ongoing achievement record try to put yourself in the next mentor's shoes. What information will they find most useful, what advice would you give them if you could talk directly to them? Write the information that you would like to receive.

WHAT HAPPENS WHEN A STUDENT DOES NOT PASS?

Some of the more common reasons for mentors to regard the act of failing a student with fear and dread are misguided beliefs regarding what their decision to fail will do. Many mentors associate failing a student with the following consequences:

- ruining the student's career
- the student will be discontinued from the programme
- destroying their mentoring reputation
- having their clinical area labelled as uncaring towards students.

If any of these were true then these would be very heavy penalties indeed for fulfilling your professional responsibility. Fortunately none of these consequences are accurate, however they are popular myths that many mentors continue to believe despite no supportive evidence. Failing a student does not result in ruining a student's career or having them kicked off a course, rather it naturally leads to a second attempt of the learning outcomes they failed to achieve.

SECOND ATTEMPTS

It is the norm in most universities that a student is automatically granted a second attempt if they have not passed their assessment at the first attempt, and this follows for the practice element of the programme. If you do fail a student then the university should already be aware of this possibility as you should have kept them fully informed of the student's progress. When the assessment document is handed in to the university then your assessment result will be recorded as a refer and the student will be offered a second attempt. The university organizes the second attempt. The second attempt may be repeated on the same placement or may be held in a different clinical area to the first attempt to allow for fresh opinions to be sought.

WHAT ABOUT MY REPUTATION AS A MENTOR?

Some mentors believe that if their student fails then this reflects badly on them. They fear being labelled as unkind, harsh or unfair. While it is true that some students may react negatively if failed on a placement, the only way that you can be justifiably labelled as a 'bad' mentor is if you have not fulfilled your professional role in this capacity.

It is very good practice after mentoring a student to reflect on you own performance as a mentor. Instead of being focused on the result the student achieved, why not assess your own performance. If you did fail a student then perhaps you might like to run through a checklist of your own performance (Box 8.1).

Box 8.1 Reflecting on your performance

	Yes/No
Did I set clear goals and objectives at the initial interview?	☐
Did I work consistently with my student so I could assess accurately?	☐
Did I inform my student as early as possible of concerns related to competence?	☐
Did I offer help, support and advice?	☐
Did I action plan?	☐
Did I provide feedback?	☐
Did I provide a timely midpoint interview?	☐
Did I document concerns, support and advice throughout the placement?	☐
Did I get help and support from my colleagues and the university?	☐
Did my student reach a competent standard?	☐
Did I fail my student?	☐

DID I FAIL?

Only you will truly know how you measure up as a mentor. The real question to ask yourself when reflecting on your own mentorship is: 'Am I competent?' Only you will know if you are able to fulfil your professional role when faced with a failing student situation? After reading this chapter you should have a good idea regarding your own standards of mentorship. Perhaps you will have reflected on a time when you may not have dealt appropriately with a student who failed to reach a competent standard. If this chapter has clarified that your performance as a mentor is what it should be then well done, keep up this great work and don't forget that you are a role model to others. If you are guilty of failing to fail then you need to address this aspect of your mentorship very quickly. Speak to a senior colleague or university lecturer on how you can improve. Never forget that ultimately, the nursing profession is relying on mentors just like you to maintain the high standards of patient care that we all aspire to.

TOP TIPS

- Set clear evidence for competence at the initial interview so that deviations from these goals can be quickly spotted.
- Talk openly with your student about their progress to ensure problems are identified honestly and addressed quickly.
- Ask the university for support, especially when developing action plans to enhance a student's capability to achieve their learning outcomes.
- Give clear and honest feedback, especially if a competent standard is unlikely to be achieved by the end of the practice placement. Failure to achieve learning outcomes should never come as a surprise.
- Consider your use of terminology, use refer rather than fail for a first attempt at an assessment.

CHAPTER 9

THE FINAL INTERVIEW

Chapter Aims

The purpose of this chapter is to explore the nature and function of the final interview. After reading the chapter you will be able to:

- Explain the purpose of the final interview.
- Identify the essential components of a successful final interview.
- Successfully conduct a final interview.

THE END OF PLACEMENT

One of the last events to take place during a student's placement is the final interview. This will always be a significant event for yourself and your student. Throughout your mentoring career it is likely that you will undertake final interviews with students at all stages of their programme; from their very first to their very last placement and every placement in between. The final interview may signify a critical moment as a student moves between modules, or progresses between years. Yet regardless of whether the placement has been of short or long duration or the student is at the beginning or end of their course, your role in the final interview will always be significant.

WHAT IS THE POINT OF A FINAL INTERVIEW?

The final interview is the final, formal stage of the assessment process for a student on practice placement. During the final interview you will have the opportunity to review the placement with the student; and this will usually include the following elements:

- finalize assessment and complete required sections in the practice assessment document
- complete the ongoing achievement record
- give final feedback to the student on their performance during the placement
- receive final feedback from the student on your performance during the placement
- debrief on significant events.

The final interview is essentially your chance to provide summarized feedback to the student on their overall performance during the placement. The feedback you provide is vital for the ongoing development of the student, whatever their stage on the programme. Your aim should therefore be to conduct a fair, honest and accurate final interview that promotes a student's self esteem and encourages them to continue to develop their skills, knowledge and professional behaviour.

> **KEY POINT**
>
> The final interview is your last chance to identify the student's strengths and areas for further development. What you say can have a major impact on their motivation for their next placement experience.

FINAL INTERVIEW CHECKLIST

You may like to consider developing a final interview checklist (Box 9.1) that can be used to guide the discussion throughout the interview. Not only will it ensure that all areas are covered, it will also ensure that all documentation is completed and that no loose ends are forgotten. Many mentors find that a checklist also helps to keep the interview within the designated timeframe as this provides a fixed agenda that both the student and mentor can use.

It is quite likely that you will have past experiences of final interviews to draw upon. Activity 9.1 provides an opportunity to reflect on your own personal experiences.

> **Box 9.1 Key features of a final interview**
>
> - Final feedback related to all learning outcomes the student has undertaken during the placement.
> - Final documentation of the practice assessment.
> - Final documentation within action plans or development plans.
> - Completion of ongoing achievement record.
> - Feedback on the student's experiences, including feedback on your performance.
> - Debrief on significant events.
> - Completion of placement timesheet or other relevant document.

Activity 9.1 Personal reflection on the final interview

Take a look at the final interview checklist in Box 9.1. Use this opportunity to reflect on your past experiences of conducting final interviews.

How many of these elements do you regularly complete?

Are there any elements that you have never done before?

If yes, what is the reason for this?

You may find it helpful to write down any factors that you feel may contribute to non-completion. As we move through this chapter we will look at the significance of each element of the final interview.

CONTENT OF THE FINAL INTERVIEW

The final interview provides you with the opportunity for completing the final assessment of the student's placement. At the final assessment you should endeavour to reflect with the student on their performance throughout the whole placement and discuss clearly your reasons for your final assessment decision. Importantly, the final assessment decision should be drawn from evidence of continual assessment that has taken place over the entire placement, and will be the culmination of all evidence over many weeks.

KEY POINT

Use open ended questions to encourage deep reflection and try to focus on specific events that have taken place during the placement. These will emphasize to the student that you have taken a keen interest in what has happened during their practice experience.

The final assessment should never be viewed as an opportunity for one-off tests or quizzes. It is simply a chance to discuss with the student how they have performed during the whole placement and reflect on the entire placement experience. By the time you reach the final assessment your student should already be aware of how they have performed during the placement and what the final assessment decision will be.

FINAL FEEDBACK TO THE STUDENT

The final interview and assessment should involve a summary of the placement as a whole. Your feedback throughout the placement should have kept the student informed of their progress towards meeting their learning outcomes. The final interview therefore will be a discussion of the evidence the student has produced, and a clear explanation of the reasons for your final assessment decision. If the student has demonstrated evidence of competence throughout the placement you should take this opportunity to discuss relevant examples and praise the student for their achievements. You could provide advice on how to develop during future practice experiences. If the student has not demonstrated evidence of competence in a learning outcome then this will be reflected in the final assessment decision. You should use the final interview to discuss why the student has not achieved competence and how they might develop this area during future placements.

KEY POINT

Don't forget to use the feedback sandwich when delivering your feedback at the end of the placement. Not only will this keep your conversation structured, it will also ensure that you remain objective in your comments.

It is very important that the final assessment decision does not contain 'surprise' assessment decisions. The feedback a student receives from you at their final interview should never be new information, or come as a shock. Remember that your feedback at this event should be a summary of feedback from the entire placement; so any feedback given at this stage should have been provided throughout the whole placement. If you find yourself giving new information at the final assessment then you have failed to provide satisfactory feedback during the placement. The impact of this is shown in Case study 9.1.

Case study **9.1** *A student speaks of her experience at final interview*

'I had a terrible experience on my last placement. My mentor called me into the office on my last day and basically said I wasn't going to pass on my drug calculations. I'm still so angry with him. I had spent 6 weeks on that ward and no-one ever mentioned that I was going to fail and then all of a sudden I'm in the office, it's my last day and I'm told 'Sorry, you're not good enough'. I just think that's cruel. If he had said something even two weeks before I could have done something about it, but telling me on the last day I had no time left to improve and so pass.'

FINAL FEEDBACK ON YOUR PERFORMANCE

The final interview should also provide your student with an opportunity to provide feedback on your performance as a mentor. You could encourage this by asking relevant questions related to the support the student has received during the placement and the feedback they received from you. Some examples are listed below to get you started.

- Did you feel welcome in the ward/clinic/unit/department – why or why not?
- Did you feel the ward/clinic/unit/department was prepared for your placement – why or why not?
- Did you have sufficient opportunities to learn – why or why not?
- How do you feel about the quality and amount of feedback you received during the placement?
- What could we/I have done to improve your experience?

Some students may feel awkward in providing feedback directly to you, especially if they believe it will affect their assessment. If you have built a good rapport with your student during the placement then honest communication between the two of you at the final interview should not be a problem. The openness of your student and willingness to provide you with feedback will provide you with feedback in itself on your skills as a mentor!

KEY POINT

You don't have to leave feedback on your performance as a mentor to the end of the placement, as this should be encouraged all the way through. However, the final discussion on your mentorship should take place at the final interview to ensure the student considers the placement as a whole.

It may be that student feedback sheds light on a problem that needs to be addressed, either personally or related to your unit or department. For this reason the feedback your student provides will be invaluable in developing your own skills as a mentor and also ensuring that the practice environment is supportive of students. You should use this feedback to take action where required. This is discussed in more detail in Chapter 14 which looks at evaluation.

COMPLETING THE PRACTICE ASSESSMENT DOCUMENT

The final interview will probably be your last opportunity to complete the practice assessment documentation. This should not be rushed as the student will be required to submit this document to their university so that the assessment can be ratified and the practice element completed. If any paperwork is outstanding or incomplete the student will need to return to your area at a later stage, causing delays in them receiving their results and unnecessary worry. For this reason you should be very clear about what and how you are required to complete the final documentation and paperwork in advance of the final interview so that you have all the resources you may require to hand. We will have the opportunity of discussing specific documentation associated with the final interview later in this chapter.

DEBRIEF ON SIGNIFICANT EVENTS

During any placement there will be events and circumstances that affect students in different ways. Remember that as an experienced nurse you will have developed coping mechanisms that you can call on when faced with difficult situations. No doubt you will have also established close working relationships with your colleagues and may turn to them for help and support when faced with the day-to-day challenges associated with delivering patient care. This isn't the case for students. While they may fit in well to your nursing team for the short period of their placement, this is not the same as developing working relationships over many years. In addition, as novices in the clinical environment, students are not only learning the science of nursing, they are learning the art as well, which includes developing the coping mechanisms they will require throughout their careers. What you may perceive as a 'normal' nursing duty, for example care of the dying patient; the student may perceive as a very traumatic event, especially if they have never experienced the situation before (see Case study 9.2).

The real skill of mentoring is in understanding your clinical environment from the student's perspective, and allowing them to express their feelings in a non-judgemental, supportive manner. While this should have been taking place throughout the placement; the final interview will probably be your last opportunity to discuss any issues or situations that may have affected the student during their practice experience.

KEY POINT

If there have been particularly difficult experiences during the placement that have impacted on your student then discuss this with a lecturer from the university. This will ensure that the student receives ongoing care and support following the placement.

Case study 9.2 *A student's first experience of a patient death*

Jenny is a first-year student and has just completed her first ever placement. In her second week of placement Jenny experienced her first patient death. She was totally unprepared for the feelings that arose while helping to lay out the body, and felt ashamed that she became tearful when speaking with the family that she had built a close rapport with. Her mentor was very friendly and tried to be supportive but Jenny never really felt she could express how she felt, especially as the other nurses in the ward seemed to be unaffected. Jenny felt a failure as a nurse, and left the placement wondering if she should continue with her training.

The final interview is a perfect opportunity to offer the student a final chance to express their feelings about the placement and any events that took place. If you are already aware of events that the student may have found challenging during the placement, then use this opportunity to discuss these specific situations. Alternatively, the student may wish to discuss an event or situation that has been important to them. Whatever the case, this is the time to ensure that the student has an opportunity to discuss openly how they feel, and learn the value of a supported debrief.

COMPLETING THE FINAL INTERVIEW AND ASSESSMENT

You should aim to complete the final interview and assessment with a student in the last week of their placement, ideally on the penultimate or final day of the placement if possible. If you complete the final interview too early there is the potential that the student's performance and motivation to learn will diminish. A final interview that takes place too early also negates the opportunity for continual assessment throughout the entire placement period; it's a bit like finishing a 100 metre race at the 80 metre mark.

LENGTH OF THE FINAL INTERVIEW

The final interview is a very important part of the placement, so it should be planned for and scheduled as a distinct event, just like all other interview situations. A final interview should never be a rushed, 5 minute event that is shoehorned into a 'space' in the day. Quite apart from limiting valuable feedback, a rushed interview will give no opportunity for a thorough debrief. If possible, the final interview should take place away from the noise and distractions of the clinical area, in a quiet and private venue such as a meeting room or office where possible. It is important that there are no distractions (Case study 9.3).

Case study 9.3 A mentor speaks about final interviews

'We are always so busy where I work, so it's hard to find the time to do an interview. I remember that once I had this poor student and we ended up doing the interview in the car on the way back to the clinic. I'm not sure to this day what I said because the traffic was so bad, and we even had to stop for petrol half-way through. I still feel really bad about it, she can't have got very much from it.'

The actual length of the interview will be somewhat dependent on the student's performance during the placement, however, in general most final interviews should be no less than 30 minutes and no more than 1 hour in length. Remember that this should be a summary of the placement, and a finalization of the paperwork, rather than a last minute assessment of learning outcomes. A final interview that lasts less than 30 minutes is unlikely to contain a thorough evaluation of either the student's experience or their performance. A final interview that lasts longer than 1 hour would suggest that there has not been enough feedback throughout the placement and that it has all been left to the end. Something to reflect upon if this happens to you!

WHO SHOULD DO THE FINAL INTERVIEW?

We have already established that the final interview is the final opportunity to complete the assessment documentation and also give and receive feedback about the placement. For this reason the final interview should be undertaken by the primary mentor of the student. If the student has been co-mentored during the placement then both mentors may choose to be present, however, if this is not possible both mentors should discuss the student's performance so that the primary mentor can provide comprehensive feedback. Case study 9.4 gives an example of one of the implications where thought has not been given as to who undertakes the final interview.

It is not just good practice that the primary mentor conducts the final interview, without their input it is highly unlikely that the assessment documentation can be finalized. For this reason, the choice of primary mentor must be based on practical considerations such as availability for the entire duration of the placement.

Case study 9.4 *A student's experience of a final interview*

Brendon is on a second year placement in a substance misuse treatment centre. He arrives on the Monday of his last week only to find that this mentor has gone on annual leave. The manager of the unit allocates him to a co-mentor for the week, and Brendon spends 2 days working with his new co-mentor, and the other day working with another nurse on the team. On the final day Brendon requests his final interview. During the interview his co-mentor looks briefly through the assessment book and then states that he is not willing to make any decisions as he has only worked with Brendon on two occasions. Brendon goes to the manager who states there is nothing he can do and suggests that Brendon return in 2 weeks when his mentor returns from leave. Brendon calls his university in panic, he is required to submit his assessment document and will be penalized for a late submission. With no other course of action Brendon is given an extension to his submission date, causing him a delay to his own holidays and a great deal of anxiety.

DECISION MAKING – BEING OBJECTIVE

It is very important that the student receives feedback on their whole performance during the placement which is based on a wide range of learning experiences, not just the opinion of the primary mentor. While the primary mentor may facilitate the final interview, ideally it should not be just their opinion that contributes to the assessment decisions or feedback.

Discussing final assessment decisions with other mentors and staff can improve the reliability of the assessment decision. While the final interview may be an opportunity to complete the assessment documentation, it should not be seen as an assessment itself. The assessment of performance should have taken place throughout the entire length of the student's placement, it should have been continuous, and the student should have received constant feedback regarding their progress towards achieving learning outcomes. While the primary mentor and co-mentor will have played a significant role in formulating learning experiences and assessing the student performance, it is also likely that the student will have undertaken learning experiences with other staff throughout the placement. These experiences will all have contributed to the assessment of the student's performance. The role of the primary and co-mentor therefore is to draw upon all this experience throughout the placement as evidence of learning progress. Objectivity comes through an overview of many experiences, not just one individual's opinion or experience.

DOCUMENTATION IN THE FINAL INTERVIEW

By the time you reach the final interview there should be a range of documented evidence that will assist you to finalize the assessment. As feedback during the student's placement should have been provided in both verbal and written form you should have a good platform for discussion and finalizing the paperwork. In general, the documentation that you will need to consider during the final interview will include the following:

- progress reports throughout the placement
- final assessment documentation
- documentation of the ongoing achievement record.

PROGRESS REPORTS THROUGHOUT THE PLACEMENT

There should be a wide variety of documented feedback from the student's placement that you can refer to at the final interview. If you reach the final interview and are faced with a blank assessment document then something has gone very, very wrong. At the very least there should be a clearly defined initial and midpoint interview, with documentation associated with the student's progress towards achieving their learning outcomes at these stages. As the primary mentor, these should be your reports and documented feedback.

There may also be action plans or development plans that may have been written to assist the student towards achieving a particular objective. These may have been documented by the student themselves, you, or other mentors that contributed to the student's learning experiences.

There may also be documentation of the student's progress in the form of learning plans, evidence of learning, or reflective exercises. All of this documentation as a whole tells the story of the placement, it provides an audit trail of what happened, what was done; evidence of what has been achieved, and evidence of what may not have been achieved. The sum total of all this documented evidence will form the basis of the final documented assessment.

FINAL ASSESSMENT DOCUMENTATION

The final interview is your opportunity to finalize the assessment documentation. Depending on the format of the assessment document this may require you to grade a student according to set criteria, or perhaps just indicate whether or not the various learning outcomes have been achieved. Whatever the format, the final assessment requires that a judgement be made. Many mentors struggle with this role, and do not feel comfortable with making the final judgement of a student's performance. However, the final interview requires you to do just that. You will be required to refer to all evidence from the student's placement to make the final judgement, perhaps by recording your signature in a box next to the specific learning outcome, or providing the student a grade for each outcome. The way the decision is to be recorded may vary according to the different types of assessment documentation, so you must make yourself aware of how the records should be completed. No matter the format, the most important aspect is that the decision you make is based on evidence of continuous assessment and does not come as a surprise to the student.

> **KEY POINT**
>
> If you need help in understanding the assessment criteria then seek advice before the final interview. Do not undertake a final interview unless you are very clear regarding the assessment mark sheets or grading schedule.

DOCUMENTING THE ONGOING ACHIEVEMENT RECORD

At the end of a student's placement you are also required to complete their ongoing achievement record. This should take the form of a documented summary of the student's placement and include evidence of the level of competency that they have achieved and the areas of competency that require further development. This means that the ongoing achievement record should be based on the feedback you provide, and match all the information that you discuss with your student at the final interview.

The ongoing achievement record will be invaluable for the student and next mentor. They will be able to use the information contained in the record to develop plans of learning for the next placement. If a student still needs to develop further competence in a particular area, this can be documented and then they and their next mentor will be provided with clear details regarding the areas that require the most support. Equally, recording evidence of achievement means that the student and next mentor can plan new experiences that extend and consolidate competence already achieved.

The ongoing achievement record also contributes to the audit trail that the sign-off mentor on the student's final placement will use when making the final assessment decision as to whether the student has achieved the required level of competence through their past and final placement. Universities are required to keep a copy of all ongoing achievement records for student nurses and midwives. The NMC requires that the documentation you provide in the ongoing achievement record should substantiate and provide evidence of the student's competence.

FAILING THE FINAL ASSESSMENT

In the last chapter we dealt with 'failure to fail' and discussed the issues associated with mentors making poor and inaccurate assessment decisions. We discussed the fact that 'failure to fail' is often the result of mentors failing to identify and assist weak students throughout the course of the placement but it is at the final interview that 'failure to fail' actually takes place. Without evidence to support the final assessment decision, mentors may be tempted to pass students who have not reached a satisfactory standard.

FAILING TO ASSESS

Previously in this chapter we have discussed the need to ensure that by the time of the final interview the assessment decision for each learning outcome should have already been reached. Sadly, many mentors still reach the final interview without having completed a continuous assessment of all learning outcomes. This creates a situation which will cause serious problems. If a mentor reaches the final interview without a firm decision regarding the assessment judgement then the fairness and accuracy of the assessment is questionable.

Typically this situation may arise when a mentor reaches the final interview and realizes that one or more learning outcomes have not been assessed throughout the placement. Very often this will not be deliberate, and is usually down to not following the assessment process throughout the placement. Under such circumstances both the mentor and student are guilty of failing to follow the assessment process. However, whatever the reason may be, a failure to assess a learning outcome creates enormous pressure on a mentor as the student will be expecting that an assessment decision is going to be made. Under such circumstances a mentor may panic, they recognize that a decision needs to be made but have little or no evidence of the student's competence. At this point a mentor has very few viable options, and none of them are attractive:

Option 1 – Action

The mentor could administer a last minute, sudden test of the student's knowledge. They may ask one or a series of questions designed to 'test' knowledge. The student's answers under these circumstances will form the basis of the mentor's assessment decision.

Option 1 – Consequence

Basing an assessment decision on a last minute, one-off test proves nothing at all. If the student manages to produce the correct answer this only provides evidence that on one occasion the student has given a correct response. It provides no evidence whatsoever that future actions or responses will also be correct. There is no reliability or validity in this judgement. Alternatively, if the student responds with an incorrect answer this is not evidence in itself that the student will be incorrect every time. So whilst a one-off assessment provides limited evidence of a student's knowledge, skill and attitude in relation to an area of practice, mentors who have not undertaken continuous assessment throughout the placement may be tempted to rely on a meaningless event to determine an assessment result. Clearly, if continuous assessment has not been undertaken this approach provides a very poor option (see Case study 9.5).

Case study 9.5 *A student speaks of her experience at final interview*

'My worst experience was during this final interview when my mentor suddenly decided to give me a drug calculation test. She said if I got the answer right she would pass me. It was like my whole life hung on that one question. In the end I was in such a state that I just guessed the answer and luckily it was right so it was a pass.'

Option 2 – Action
The mentor could choose to pass the student on the learning outcome with no specific evidence of their achievement. A mentor who is under pressure to reach a decision with no evidence on which to base that decision may be tempted to pass the student anyway on the basis that they have not heard anything to say the student is not competent. At the time it may seem like the best option, and while it may not be accurate, valid or reliable, it is also unlikely to cause any conflict. A mentor may be tempted to justify this course of action based on a belief that if the decision is incorrect then 'someone else' will pick it up with the student at a later stage.

Option 2 – Consequence
Passing a student as achieving a learning outcome without evidence, out of guilt or wishing to avoid conflict is a serious failure of a mentor's professional accountability and responsibility. Hoping that 'someone else' will review the assessment at a later date creates serious problems for any future mentor, and denies the student the help and support they require. If the non-evidenced-based pass occurs on the student's final placement, this decision becomes a sign off for qualification.

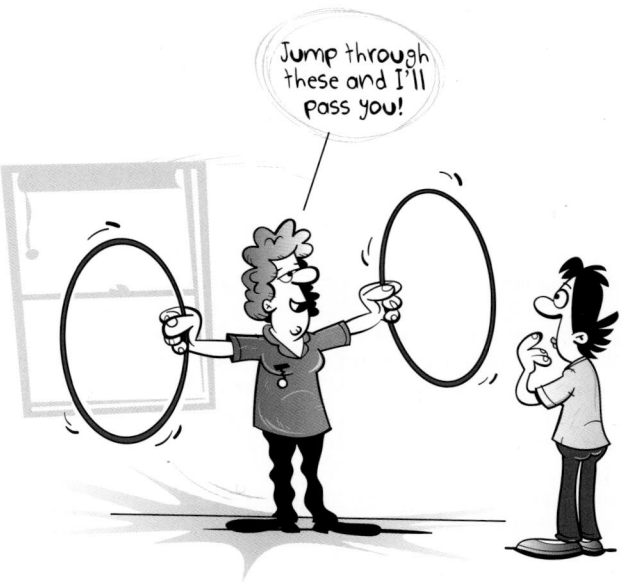

Option 3 – Action

The mentor could choose to fail the student based on the fact that there is no evidence of achievement. Particularly in assessment documents where the only option is to record if the student has achieved or not achieved the learning outcome this approach could be appealing as a course of action. In this circumstance the mentor may decide that if they cannot confirm the student has 'achieved' then the only alternative is 'not achieved'.

Option 3 – Consequence

While this decision may be the most 'technically' correct option based on the circumstances, very few mentors would be willing to fail a student based on their failure to assess a learning outcome. This action is likely to cause conflict and a student could appeal the decision at the university as due process has not been followed as they have not been given an opportunity to demonstrate competence.

Option 4 – Action

The mentor could choose to do no assessment at all. When a mentor realizes they have not assessed a learning outcome they may feel that the only option open to them is to avoid the assessment altogether. In other words, if they haven't got the evidence to support an assessment decision they may choose to just not complete the assessment paperwork. Such a situation will no doubt cause conflict as the student will be expecting an assessment decision. Unless they have been informed otherwise, they will be expecting to pass their learning outcomes. They will not be expecting to hear that their mentor has forgotten to assess them and is therefore unwilling to make a decision at all.

Option 4 – Consequence

While it might be very tempting to do nothing if you have failed to or forgotten to undertake assessment, this does cause serious repercussions. The whole point of the student undertaking a practice placement is so that they may be provided with the types of learning experiences that allow for assessment of competence. If a student reaches the end of a placement and competence has not been assessed this does raise the question as to what they and you have been doing during the placement. The likely outcome is that the student will be deferred by the university and be given a further opportunity to be assessed on the learning outcome either by returning to this placement or undertaking it on another placement. If this is their final placement then this will delay their completion of the programme.

WHICH OPTION?

While it is quite clear that none of these options are attractive, it is also clear that one option will have to be taken – even if it is by default. A mentor in this situation would find themselves having to make a choice between the best of the only options available to them. Quite clearly they cannot justify passing a student based on poor evidence, or passing a student based on no evidence. Options 1 and 2 are therefore in total contradiction with their professional accountability. This leaves only options 3 or 4, failing the student or doing no assessment. While neither of these options is ideal, they are also the only options left. In these circumstances a mentor should contact the university and a link lecturer immediately for advice and support. Being honest about the circumstances is vital here; the support and advice you receive will prevent an unsatisfactory situation from becoming even worse. Keep in mind that the only two options open to you will by necessity cause the student some degree of distress, and there is a high potential for conflict under such circumstances. Contacting the university will not only provide support for you but also ensure the student is supported through this time.

THE FAILING MENTOR

It should be quite clear that failure to assess a learning outcome during a practice placement is a situation that should be avoided at all costs. It is far too late to realize at the final interview that vital assessments have been missed. As we have seen, there are no good options for mentors who find themselves in this situation, as each possible course of action will have serious consequences for them and the student.

The best way to avoid this error is to conduct a thorough initial interview where all learning outcomes are discussed and plans put in place to undertake appropriate learning experiences. In Chapter 5 we discussed a 'checklist' for the initial interview that ensured thorough plans can be made. Likewise, in Chapter 7 we identified that at the midpoint interview there should have been a thorough review of progress on all learning outcomes. If progress is not being made or evidence of progress is not available then this should be picked up and planned for in the second half of the placement. If these two formal stages of the interview process are not satisfactory then learning outcomes can be missed. Situations such as this reflect poor mentoring practice, and serious failings of a mentor's professional accountability and responsibility.

ENDING ON A HIGH NOTE

At the final interview you have an ideal opportunity to encourage the student to continue to develop both personally and professionally. As you reflect together on the placement you will have the opportunity of hearing from the student the events and circumstances they have valued the most during the course of their placement. Perhaps they were encouraged by something that you said or did that has made a positive lasting impression. Be proud of yourself for these achievements, as that student will reap the benefit of your excellent mentorship. Perhaps there were events and circumstances that the student found challenging that they wished to ask your advice and support about before they leave. Be proud of yourself for these achievements, as your student clearly appreciates your professionalism and values your experience. Perhaps there were events and circumstances that you could have improved on, instances where mentoring has been less than satisfactory. Do not be too proud to acknowledge that mistakes and errors can be learned from and improved in future learning experiences.

REFLECTION ON YOUR EXPERIENCE

While the final interview might signal the end of the placement for the student, it is not quite the end for you. The end of a student's placement provides you with an opportunity to self-evaluate your mentoring performance. We will look at strategies you can use for this in Chapter 14.

IMPROVING YOUR OWN STANDARD OF MENTORING

When you are the mentor of a student, there are effectively two people being assessed. While it is true that you are assessing the student; your own ability, skill and professionalism as a mentor is also under scrutiny. At the end of each placement experience you have a valuable opportunity to reflect on your mentoring performance. This opportunity should never be taken lightly or wasted. Seize this chance to reflect on yourself and develop as a mentor. Improve on the areas that are weak, and strengthen those which serve you well. Not only will you reap the benefit, but so will all students who are privileged to benefit from your mentoring in future.

 TOP TIPS

- Try to plan for the final interview and assessment by blocking out time in the day or recording the event in the ward diary.
- Arrange for the co-mentor to be present during the final interview if possible.
- Resist the temptation to administer last minute tests or quizzes as the assessment decision should already be clear.
- Ask the student for their feedback on your performance as a mentor.

CHAPTER 10

THE ROLE OF THE SIGN-OFF MENTOR

Chapter Aims

The purpose of this chapter is to gain an understanding of the role of the sign-off mentor. After reading this chapter you will be able to:

- List the criteria for becoming a sign-off mentor.
- Appreciate the accountability of the sign-off mentor to the NMC when making the final assessment decision.
- Appreciate the role of the ongoing achievement record in assisting the sign-off mentor to make their confirmation of a student's proficiency at the end of their programme.

WHAT IS A SIGN-OFF MENTOR?

The sign-off mentor role was introduced by the NMC in their *Standards to Support Learning and Assessment in Practice* in 2006. It is this role that has probably caused the most concern for mentors as it makes explicit the mentor's accountability to the NMC in signing off a student's proficiencies at the end of their programme. In reality a mentor has always been accountable for their decisions but the creation of a separate role has highlighted the significance of signing off a student as being ready, from a practice perspective, to register with the NMC.

A sign-off mentor is a mentor who has met additional criteria and who will make the judgement as to whether or not a student has achieved the required standards of proficiency for safe and effective practice for entry to the NMC register (NMC, 2008). In addition they must be designated as a sign-off mentor on the local register of mentors. A sign-off mentor must be on the same part and field of practice as that the student is intending to enter. They have been mandatory for all students commencing NMC approved programmes from September 2007. The role of the sign-off mentor differs slightly for different parts of the register (see Table 10.1).

Table 10.1 When is a sign-off mentor required?

Programme	When a sign-off mentor is required
Pre-registration Nursing	Only for final placement
Pre-registration Midwifery	At each progression point across the whole programme
Specialist Practice Programmes that lead to a recordable qualification on the NMC register	For the whole programme or it can be a Practice Teacher if required by the commissioners of the programme
Overseas Nursing Programme	For the whole programme
Return to Practice Programme	For the whole programme

KEY POINT

A sign-off mentor is currently only required for pre-registration nursing students on their final placement. If you don't have students on their final placement you don't require a sign-off mentor.

HOW DO I BECOME A SIGN-OFF MENTOR?

To become a sign-off mentor you must already be a mentor on a local register of mentors and demonstrate that you have met the additional criteria to be a sign-off mentor. Box 10.1 summarizes these and we will look at each of these criteria in turn.

Clinical currency and capability in the field in which the student is being assessed

All registrants have a professional responsibility to keep themselves up-to-date. If you have an annual appraisal you can use this as evidence of your currency and capability. If you have not had an appraisal in the last year you should make an appointment with your line manager to arrange one as soon as possible. If there is a personal or professional development plan ensure that the agreed actions are being implemented. You will also have confirmed to the NMC every three years, by completing a notification of practice form, that you have completed the required hours of learning activity relevant to your practice. However, if you change your place of work (e.g. moving from a medical ward to an Intensive Care Unit) it may be that your clinical currency and capability is lacking in that

> **Box 10.1 Additional criteria to be a sign-off mentor**
>
> A sign-off mentor must have:
> - Clinical currency and capability in the field in which the student is being assessed.
> - A working knowledge of current programme requirements, practice assessment strategies and relevant changes in education and practice for the student they are assessing.
> - An understanding of the NMC registration requirements and the contribution they make to the achievement of these requirements.
> - An in-depth understanding of their accountability to the NMC for the decision they must make to pass or fail a student when assessing proficiency requirements at the end of a programme.
> - Been supervised on at least three occasions for signing off proficiency by an existing sign-off mentor.
>
> (NMC, 2008 p. 21)

particular speciality such that you would be unable to mentor a student in that area with confidence. In this situation you would need to gain experience in that area and discuss with your manager through the annual appraisal process when you have the appropriate level of competence to mentor a student. Now complete Activity 10.1.

> **Activity 10.1 Evidence of clinical currency and capability**
>
> Record below the date of your last appraisal
>
> Which part of the register/field of practice are you registered for?
>
> List below the action points from your personal/professional development plan and any additional activities you have undertaken in the last year.
> 1
> 2
> 3
> 4
> 5

In order to sign-off a student you must be on the same part of the register and field of practice as that of the student you will be mentoring. This means that if you are registered as a mental health nurse you can only sign-off students on the mental health branch programme. If you hold a second registration you cannot sign-off a student from that branch unless you can demonstrate clinical currency and capability in that field of practice.

A working knowledge of current programme requirements, practice assessment strategies and relevant changes in education and practice for the student they are assessing

This aspect of the role requires you to have an understanding of the programme your students are on. Attendance at annual mentor updates should give you a good feel of the above requirements for your students. You don't need to know the programme in detail but should have an understanding of:

- The different modules in the programme, particularly the modules students will be on when they come to your area for their practice experience.
- The different types of placement experiences the students will have during the course of their programme.
- The assessment documentation and processes for supporting a failing student.
- Any changes to the programme that have implications for you as a mentor.
- The role of the ongoing achievement record (OAR) in helping you make the final assessment decision.

An understanding of the NMC registration requirements and the contribution mentors make to the achievement of these requirements

The NMC sets the standards of proficiency for the programmes they approve. These can be obtained from the NMC website under the education section. All students are required to meet the standards of proficiency through completion of the programme that has been approved by the NMC. The NMC website can be accessed at www.nmc-uk.org.

All pre-registration nursing students are required to complete 2300 hours of theory and 2300 hours of practice, which the university has to confirm that a student has completed to the NMC before the student can register with them. As 50% of a student's programme is spent in practice, mentors play a significant role in facilitating the overall programme. Most universities will require mentors to confirm the number of hours a student has completed during their practice placement. It is very important therefore that these are accurate and any absences that the student has while on placement are recorded on the attendance record but it is also important that you inform the university directly as well. If a student asks to make up any missed time while on their placement with you this may be possible but check with your university and always inform them that this has been arranged otherwise they will have no evidence that the student has been sick or absent.

Progressing on the pre-registration programme

Pre-registration programmes have progression points. These are points along the programme where the student is required to meet certain requirements set by the NMC before they can continue on the programme. In nursing the first progression point is at the end of year one. Students must have completed the correct number of hours (767 hours each of theory and practice) and passed all their theory and practice assessments within 12 weeks of completing their first year in order to progress to the second year. As a mentor it is your responsibility to ensure that their practice assessment documentation is complete including their OAR and that their attendance record is signed. This information will be passed to the assessment/progression board at the university who will make the final decision as to whether the student meets the criteria to progress on the programme. Currently, the next progression point is at the end of the programme. Undertake Activity 10.2 if you support students on other programmes leading to registration with the NMC.

Activity 10.2 NMC requirements for other programmes leading to registration

If you have students on other programmes that lead to registration on the NMC register, e.g. Overseas Nursing Programme or Return to Practice, Midwifery, Specialist Community Public Health Nursing, Nurse Prescribing find out what the NMC registration requirements are and make a note of them.

An in-depth understanding of their accountability to the NMC for the decision they must make to pass or fail a student when assessing proficiency requirements at the end of a programme

As a mentor you are always professionally responsible and accountable to the NMC for the assessment decisions that you make. However, as a sign-off mentor you are also professionally responsible and accountable to the NMC for the *final decision* regarding whether a student has successfully completed all the practice requirements of their programme prior to their entry to the professional register.

Your student will have a section in their practice assessment document or OAR where you will be required to sign that the student has met all the practice requirements of the programme. This will be taken into account by the university's assessment board where they will make the final decision as to whether the student has met all the required criteria to pass the programme and join the professional register. Only the sign-off mentor can make the final judgements on a student's competency in practice. The university makes judgements on the student's achievement of the theoretical elements of the programme and assures itself that both practice and theory elements have been met as well as completion of the 2300 hours of theory and 2300 hours of practice. It is the university's responsibility to inform the NMC that the student has met the requirements of the programme which has been approved by the NMC and also to sign a declaration in support of the student's self-declaration that they are of good health and good character.

This means that if you sign-off a student who is not competent but has met all other requirements of the programme they will be able to register as a nurse. Equally if you do not believe that a student is competent, and document the appropriate evidence, then that student will not be able to register as a nurse. In the latter case the university will usually give the student a further attempt to achieve any outstanding practice learning outcomes by returning for a further period in practice.

KEY POINT

Only a sign-off mentor can decide whether a student is fit for practice. The university decides whether a student is fit for the award.

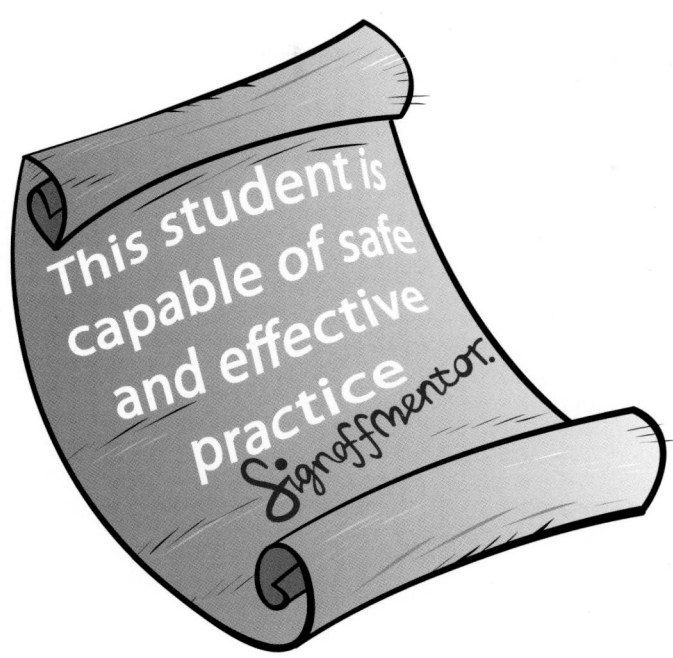

The issue of whether to fail a student or not is what taxes mentors most. If you have any doubt at all about a student's competence then you must not sign the student off. However, you cannot simply refuse to sign the student off without evidence. There must be clear documentation as to your reasons for not signing the student off which will also include evidence that:

- concerns about the student's competence/professional behaviour were raised during the course of their placement, discussed with the student and documented
- an action plan was put in place and documented detailing:
  - what the student was required to do in order to improve their competence/professional behaviour
  - the support to be given

- the time frame in which this would take place
- clearly set out measurable outcomes for the student to demonstrate at the end of that time frame.

If the above is not demonstrated then the university will judge that due process has not been followed and the student will be offered a further first attempt at their final practice assessment.

If you are in any doubt or have any concerns, talk to colleagues in practice who have worked with the student and ask for advice from the lecturers at your student's university. Wherever possible always seek advice as early as possible so there is time to put in place a plan to manage your concerns.

Chapter 8 looks in more detail at the failing student and it is recommended that you read this chapter to further understand your responsibility and accountability with regards to failing a student. Now look at Activity 10.3.

Activity 10.3

You have been Sarah's mentor during her final 12 week placement. At her midpoint interview you discussed your concerns regarding her poor communication and organizational skills, specifically poor handovers of patients to staff, which lacked essential information about the patients, failing to keep staff informed when the condition of patients changed, poor record keeping in patients' care plans and an inability to prioritize care when caring for a group of patients. An action plan was put in place and although her communication skills have improved her ability to prioritize care is still poor. Sarah is well-liked by the staff and desperate to qualify as she is a single parent with two children.

What are the implications if you sign her off?

What are the implications if you don't sign her off?

Answer to Activity 10.3

If you sign Sarah off there is little doubt that Sarah will be very grateful to you and you will have avoided giving her bad news. However, if she is unable to prioritize the care of her patients, patients could be put at risk. While this is a skill which can be developed over time you do not know what support will be available to Sarah in her first post. As a registered nurse she must be capable of safe and effective practice without supervision and it is possible that she could be placed in a position as a newly qualified nurse where she is left in charge of a group of patients or even a ward where there is limited or no support. Would you feel confident that she could cope and that the patients in her care would come to no harm? Remember your first duty is to the patient not to Sarah.

If you don't sign Sarah off you will be faced with what will be a difficult final interview with a distressed student. However, as you had already discussed your concerns with her at the midpoint interview and given her feedback since the final decision this should not come as a surprise to her. As this is her first attempt she will be offered a further attempt by her university and this will give her the opportunity to further develop her competence in this area. More importantly you will not have placed patients at risk.

Something that may have helped you in making your final assessment decision would have been comments made by previous mentors on the student's performance and progress. This record of mentors' comments is known as the OAR. If it had highlighted concerns regarding Sarah's communication or organizational skills this would have been further evidence that you could use to support your decision. We will look more at the OAR later in this chapter.

Been supervised on at least three occasions for signing off proficiency by an existing sign-off mentor

Before you are designated as a sign-off mentor on the mentor register you must be supervised by a mentor who is already designated as a sign-off mentor on a mentor register whilst undertaking the signing off of the final proficiencies for a student.

On pre-registration nursing programmes this means that you will require access to three students on their final placement of their programme. For most mentors in an acute hospital setting this is less of a problem as there will be a steady flow of final placement students being placed within the hospital. If your local university has two intakes a year there will be opportunities twice a year; however, if your university only has one intake a year then this could potentially take three years to accomplish. However, for placement areas that do not take final placement students very often, such as nursing homes, the community and specialist placement areas this could take significantly longer.

Due to these challenges the NMC decided in 2010 that the first two of the sign-offs can now be undertaken through other means such as using simulation, role play, OSCEs etc. Your university will have agreed a process for these alternative approaches with your organization. However, the third sign-off must be with an actual student on an NMC approved programme.

KEY POINT

Undertaking three sign-offs could take years if you rarely take final placement students. Contact the university to explore how this could be achieved using alternative approaches for two of them or whether it is appropriate for you to be a sign-off mentor.

PREPARING FOR YOUR ROLE AS SIGN-OFF MENTOR

There is no specific requirement for a mentor to undertake any additional study in order to become a sign-off mentor. The first wave of sign-off mentors would have been identified by their managers to ensure that there was a critical mass in place. All new sign-off mentors will need to demonstrate that they have met the criteria listed in Box 10.1. You can complete a self-assessment at the end of this chapter to reassure yourself that you have met all these criteria.

SUPPORTING OTHERS

As a sign-off mentor you are also expected to support colleagues who are acting as mentors to students and require advice or support in relation to the mentoring and assessment process. For example:

- supporting a new mentor through the mentoring process with their first student
- giving advice to a mentor on managing the failing student
- helping a mentor and student to develop an action plan where concerns have been raised.

It is also possible that you may be asked to act as what is often called a 'long arm' sign-off mentor. A long arm sign-off mentor can be used when a student is on a final placement where there is no sign-off mentor available. Long-arm mentoring requires a regular commitment from the sign-off mentor. You will need to:

- be present at the initial and midpoint interview
- ask to see the student's OAR at the start of the placement in order to identify any areas of concern that have been raised by previous mentors and not addressed that will need to be addressed within this final placement
- meet with the student on a regular basis in order that they have the one hour a week protected time with you as stipulated by the NMC (discussed below)

- undertake the final assessment of proficiencies with the student at the end of their placement.

It is important to note that if you undertake this role you are the person responsible for signing off the student at the end of their placement not the mentor that they have been working with.

MAKING TIME TO MEET WITH YOUR STUDENT

All mentors are expected to supervise their students (directly or indirectly) whilst giving direct care for 40% of their time on placement. However, a student on their final placement is also expected to have an additional *one hour* a week protected time to spend with their sign-off mentor. This does not have to be exactly one hour per week. Where a student is identified early in the placement as requiring additional support and development this time might be frontloaded into the placement with less time given later in the placement.

Making time during a busy work day is likely to be challenging at times and you will need to negotiate this protected time with your manager, for example, negotiating a smaller case load on the day you have planned to meet with your student. What is essential is to plan the time in your diaries. This will commit you both to a specific day and time and allow colleagues to plan around you if required. Consider whether there is a specific day of the week and/or time that is easier for you both to meet up and have this protected time.

HOW DO I USE MY ONE HOUR A WEEK?

The time is to be used to reflect and give feedback to the student on their performance and very importantly to document assessment decisions as well as developing action plans where there are concerns regarding the student's progress. Through regular meetings there should then be no surprise to the student on your final assessment decision. Chapters 6 and 7 in this book will be helpful in guiding you on giving feedback and Chapter 8 will help in how to manage the student who is not making the expected level of progress.

Key to making the best use of these sessions is preparation. For each meeting it will be helpful if you:
1. Reflect on what the student has done well.
2. Reflect on the areas that the student needs to improve upon.

3. Identify the evidence (examples of actions by the student with dates, feedback from other staff) that you will bring to the meeting to support points 1 and 2 above.

4. Look at any action points that were agreed at the last meeting and ensure that you completed any that were your responsibility.

Remember to document these meetings in the student's practice documentation so that there is an official record of these meetings but also so that there is a clear audit trail leading to your final decision.

THE ONGOING ACHIEVEMENT RECORD

The OAR was introduced by the NMC in their *Standards to Support Learning and Assessment in Practice* in 2006 but was originally called the Student Passport. It became a requirement for students on all NMC approved programmes that started from September 2007.

The OAR is held by the student and taken from placement to placement so that mentors can make judgements on the student's progress. While the format may vary between different universities it will have areas in it for the mentor to comment on the student's performance and behaviour, and may have headings such as:

● Strengths
● Development needs
● Concerns.

As confidential information is being shared between mentors all students are required to sign a form at the university at the start of their programme consenting to the sharing of these data. If they refuse to consent then they would be unable to meet the requirements of the programme and would be unable to continue on the programme. A copy of the OAR must be kept by the university.

The OAR is essential for the sign-off mentor as they must use it to confirm that the student has maintained ongoing competence throughout their programme and that where any concerns have been expressed that these have been addressed.

As a mentor what you write is very important. Remember that the student's sign-off mentor on their last placement will be making their final assessment decision based on what you and other mentors have written. This means that if you write a glowing report but in fact have some concerns about your student that you do not document the sign-off mentor will be unaware of this. Let's take a look at an example of a student's OAR to see what the implications are of what you write (Activity 10.4).

Activity 10.4

Joe is a mental health student who has been well-liked on his first-year placement. He is keen to learn and always willing to help out. His knowledge of medications however is very poor but the mentor thinks that as he is a first year student he has plenty of time to improve. Below are her comments in his OAR.

Ongoing achievement record

Strengths

Joe is a good communicator, is motivated and willing to learn.

Areas for Development

Joe would like to gain more experience in acute mental health placements and improve his reflective skills.

Concerns

More knowledge needed on medications.

How useful do you think these comments will be for the mentor on the next placement in identifying Joe's learning needs?

Comments on Activity 10.4

There is a distinct lack of detail here. The impression one gains is that Joe appears to be a willing student but does that mean he is competent? The need for Joe to gain more acute mental health experience is not within the power of a mentor and so not very useful. The need to improve his reflective skills is probably something that the university may help with although a mentor can ask Joe to reflect on his experiences and discuss them with them to help develop these skills.

The mentor has documented their concern regarding Joe's knowledge of medication management but the comment lacks any detail. Does Joe need to improve his knowledge of specific types of drugs, how they work, or how to do drug calculations? It will be difficult for the next mentor to determine exactly what their focus should be. Box 10.2 shows how the mentor could have written Joe's OAR in a way that would be more helpful for future mentors and the final sign-off mentor.

The OAR in Box 10.2 will be far more helpful to the next mentor and final sign-off mentor. The mentor on the next placement will be able to draw up an action plan that sets out how Joe will be given the opportunity to practise both drawing up injections and his injection technique. At the

Box 10.2 Ongoing achievement record

Strengths

Joe's strengths include the ability to understand various aspects relating to people suffering from dementia, for example their inability to express themselves and poor memory, etc.

Joe has effective communication skills. He has integrated well with the nursing team and shows great ability to liaise with other members of the multidisciplinary teams. He is able to document patient care concisely and accurately under supervision and can be relied upon to always inform staff about changes in a client's condition.

Joe has shown enthusiasm to learn new skills, is always punctual and professionally presented.

Areas for improvement

Joe has found medication management challenging. In particular he has found it difficult to draw up injections as he hasn't developed the dexterity required and is very nervous when giving injections to clients. He requires more practice in both these areas to become more technically competent in this skill.

Concerns

There are no concerns regarding Joe's performance on this placement. He met the required level of competence in all his learning outcomes.

end of this placement the mentor should record the progress Joe has made on his injection technique and whether any further improvements are required. The sign-off mentor will look at Joe's practice assessment documents and OARs to see whether Joe was given the opportunity to practise his injection technique and whether Joe has made the required improvement. It is therefore very important that each mentor records progress made against any areas for development or concerns that have been raised on previous placements.

It is sometimes difficult to distinguish the difference between areas for development and areas of concern. Areas for development are where a student may have met the required level of competence for their stage on the programme but still needs more practice to deliver the skill with ease. In Joe's case he could draw up injections and give them safely but was very slow and his nervousness was apparent which could impact on the confidence of the patient in the care he gave. Areas for development could also include areas that could stretch a student who is doing well that bit further. For example, Joe appears to have a good understanding of clients with dementia and it could be suggested that he explores this area in more detail by reading the Department of Health's National Dementia Strategy which is available on their website at www. doh.gov.uk.

Areas of concern relate to aspects of a student's performance or behaviour that have not improved during a student's placement despite discussion with the student and an action plan being put in place to address these concerns. They may or may not relate to specific learning outcomes to be achieved. Where concerns are documented there should also be evidence of actions taken and the student's progress against agreed actions.

USING THE STUDENT'S OAR TO MAKE AN ASSESSMENT DECISION

As a sign-off mentor you are expected to use the student's OAR to help you make the final assessment decision as to whether or not the student has maintained their competency. You must also check to see if any concerns have been raised during any of their placements and whether these have been addressed since the student's last progression point. For nursing students your focus is on their progress since the end of year one which was their last progression point.

You must ask for the student's OAR at the start of the placement in order that you can identify whether any concerns have been raised and how they have been addressed. Ask yourself:

- Is the record complete for all placements?
- Have any concerns been raised?
- If yes, is there evidence that an action plan was put in place?
- Is there recorded evidence that the student has made the required improvement set out in the action plan?
- Is there evidence that the student has passed their learning outcomes/ proficiencies/objectives for all previous placements?

If you answer 'no' for any of the above you will need to discuss this further with the link lecturer for your area or the student's personal tutor to identify why there may be inconsistencies or incomplete areas in the student's record.

SELF-ASSESSMENT – AM I READY?

If you have read through this chapter and completed all the activities you should feel ready to consider taking on the role of a sign-off mentor but as a quick recap complete the check list at the end of this chapter to reassure yourself that you meet all the required criteria (Table 10.2).

Table 10.2 Meeting the criteria to be a sign-off mentor			
Criteria for a sign-off mentor	Yes	No	Actions to take if No
Are you on a live Register of Mentors?			If this is because you haven't attended an update in the last year – attend a mentor update and inform the holder of the live register. If for another reason discuss with your link lecturer
Do you have clinical currency and capability in the field in which the student is being assessed?			Discuss your CPD* needs with your line manager
Do you have working knowledge of current programme requirements, practice assessment strategies and relevant changes in education and practice for the student you are assessing?			Attend a mentor update. Discuss with the link lecturer from the university
Do you understand the NMC registration requirements and the contribution you will make to the achievement of these requirements?			Discuss with the link lecturer from the university
Do you have an in-depth understanding of your accountability to the NMC for the decision you must make to pass or fail a student when assessing proficiency requirements at the end of a programme?			Read the NMCs Standards *to Support Learning and Assessment in Practice* (2008) section 3.2.5
Have you completed three sign-offs with the last of an actual student and supervised by a sign-off mentor?			Arrange to undertake these with a sign-off mentor
*CPD, continuing professional development.			

TOP TIPS

- Not all placements require a sign-off mentor, check with your university to see if it is appropriate for you to be one.
- It will take time to undertake your three supervised sign-offs so start planning well-ahead.
- Accurate completion of the OAR is vital whether you are a mentor or a sign-off mentor.

CHAPTER 11

MENTORING STUDENTS WITH DISABILITIES

Chapter Aims

The purpose of this chapter is to explore your role as a mentor in supporting a student with a disability(ies). After reading this chapter you will be able to:

- Understand what the Disability Discrimination Act (1995) means for you as a mentor.
- Define what disability is and appreciate the implications of different models of disability.
- Develop the skills to respond to a student who discloses a disability.
- Understand how reasonable adjustments can be implemented for a student.
- Consider how to support and assess a disabled student in a way that is fair and transparent.

INTRODUCTION

Before we start let's get a feel of what your thoughts are about disabled students by completing Activity 11.1.

Hopefully you have ticked all of the boxes. This is because the answer is that none of these impairments would automatically prevent someone from applying to become a nurse, regardless of their branch. Disability legislation requires that a course design must aim to ensure it is accessible to students with disabilities and anticipate and remove potential barriers.

The NMC is quite clear that neither significant health impairments nor a disability would necessarily prevent someone from becoming a nurse. Each applicant who declares a disability is considered on an individual basis to identify what, if any, reasonable adjustments would be required to help them undertake the programme and achieve the competence standards required. The focus is always on whether or not a student will

Activity 11.1 Entry into nursing

Below is a list of common disabilities. Which of the following impairments/disabilities do you believe would *not* prevent someone from applying to become a student nurse? (Place a tick where you believe that the impairment would not prevent someone from being able to become a nurse within the specified field of practice.)

Disability	Adult Nurse	Mental Health Nurse	Child Health Nurse	Learning Disability Nurse
Bipolar affective disorder				
Diabetes				
Dyscalculia				
Dyslexia				
Epilepsy				
Hearing impairment				
HIV				
Multiple sclerosis				
Partial limb loss (hand/arm)				
Partial limb loss (foot/leg)				
Visual impairment				

be able to practice safely and effectively. We will explore reasonable adjustments in more detail later as these will directly involve you as a mentor.

MODELS OF DISABILITY

Models of disability offer different ways of looking at disability and therefore influence how you might respond to a disabled person. The two significant models of disability are the medical model and the social model.

THE MEDICAL MODEL OF DISABILITY

The medical model sees a disability as the individual's problem, with the disabled person dependent on others and either needing to be cured or cared for. In this model the focus is on the negatives: what the disabled person cannot do (walk, read text, hear, etc.).

Under the Disability Discrimination Act (DDA) (1995) a disability is 'a physical or mental impairment which has a substantial and long-term adverse effect on a person's ability to carry out normal day-to-day activities'. A disability can be due to a whole range of impairments which can be usefully grouped under a number of headings. Box 11.1 lists those that are now used on the Universities and Colleges Admissions Service (UCAS) forms for those applying to a university.

Box 11.1 Disability categories

All applicants to a university will be asked to complete a section on the application form where they are offered the opportunity to declare whether they have a disability or impairment. The categories used are:

- No disability.
- You have a social/communication impairment such as Asperger's syndrome/other autistic spectrum disorder.
- You are blind or have a serious visual impairment uncorrected by glasses.
- You are deaf or have a serious hearing impairment.
- You have a long-standing illness or health condition such as cancer, HIV, diabetes, chronic heart disease, or epilepsy.
- You have a mental health condition, such as depression, schizophrenia or anxiety disorder.
- You have a specific learning difficulty such as dyslexia, dyspraxia or attention deficit hyperactivity disorder.
- You have physical impairment or mobility issues, such as difficulty using your arms or using a wheelchair or crutches.
- You have a disability, impairment or medical condition that is not listed above.
- You have two or more impairments and/or disabling medical conditions.

Following an amendment to the Act in 2005 people with human immunodeficiency virus (HIV) infection, cancer or multiple sclerosis also meet the definition of having a disability.

THE SOCIAL MODEL

The social model was developed by disabled people in response to the medical model which is seen as segregating disabled people from the rest of society. With the social model, disability is not an individual's problem rather it is a social issue with the environment disabling the individual. Barriers that can prevent disabled people from participating in society include:

- attitudinal barriers
- physical barriers
- policies or procedural barriers
- communication barriers.

For example, on a busy ward, a hearing person telephone has not been designed to be adjustable for a person with a hearing impairment and so will prevent that person from answering the phone. Your attitudes to disabled students will be influenced by your culture, background, education, and ethnicity. As a nurse many of the patients you care for will have an impairment that will be viewed as a disability. It will therefore be easy to fall into the trap of seeing a disabled student as a person needing to be cared for (the medical model) and requiring them to 'fit in' within the existing structures and processes. If you subscribe to the social model your approach will be very different as your focus will be on removing the barriers that prevent your student from participating fully in their placement. The social model is linked to ideas of inclusivity and widening participation, looking at ways to overcome challenges and move forward.

DISABILITY AND THE LAW

There are a number of legal requirements that you need to be aware of in relation to disabled students. The key ones are:

- The DDA (1995) which sets out a legal framework which protects disabled people from discrimination and sets out the duties that organizations have towards disabled people.
- The Special Educational Needs and Disability Act (SENDA) (2001), which amended part 4 of the DDA to prohibit discrimination in the education sector.

- The DDA (2005), which was an amendment that requires all public bodies (e.g. the NHS and education sector) to actively promote disability equality and produce a Disability Equality Scheme. It also extended the definition of disability to include cancer, HIV infection and multiple sclerosis and no longer required mental health difficulties to be 'clinically well recognized'.

You do need to understand your responsibilities as a mentor and should have attended sessions in your workplace around equality and diversity which would include both the role of the organization and your own in relation to disability legislation. To help you the following sections summarize the main duties an organization has under the DDA which fall under the following headings:

- direct discrimination
- disability-related discrimination
- victimization
- harassment
- reasonable adjustments.

DIRECT DISCRIMINATION

This means treating a person less favourably than another person who is not disabled, solely on the grounds of their disability. This often occurs due to stereotypical assumptions or prejudice, for example, turning down an applicant to a nursing course because they have a disability even though they have met all the admission criteria. Equally, if a hospital refused to allow students who were deaf or dyslexic, for example, to have placements with them that would also be direct discrimination.

DISABILITY-RELATED DISCRIMINATION

In this case discrimination occurs for a disability-related reason, whereby the disabled person is treated less favourably for a reason related to their disability rather than the disability itself and it is not possible to show that that reason is justified. For example, failing a student in their practice assessment because they write slowly due to their disability would be disability-related discrimination, as there is no requirement within the competence standards for students to be able to complete patient/client documentation within a specified time-frame.

VICTIMIZATION

Victimization is unlawful under the DDA and relates to someone being victimized who makes or supports an allegation of disability discrimination regardless of whether that person is themselves disabled or not.

HARASSMENT

The harassment provision protects the disabled person from behaviour that creates an environment that the person perceives as hostile, intimidating, degrading, humiliating or offensive. This could be, for example, making jokes or derogatory remarks about their disability, blocking wheelchair access or interfering with any special support equipment they use.

REASONABLE ADJUSTMENTS

The DDA requires reasonable adjustments to be made. There is no definitive list of what constitutes a reasonable adjustment as these will depend on the type of disability, how the individual manages it, and the nature of the work activities the disabled person is involved in. Examples particularly relevant to students are:

- making adjustments to premises
- altering a student's hours of working or training
- assigning a student to a different placement
- allowing the student to be absent during working or training hours for rehabilitation, assessment or treatment
- giving, or arranging for, training or mentoring (whether for the disabled person or any other person)
- acquiring or modifying equipment
- modifying instructions or reference manuals
- modifying procedures for testing or assessment
- providing a reader or interpreter
- providing supervision or other support.

However, consideration will need to be given to the practicality of the adjustments, the health and safety implications for the student and others as well as the financial or other resources of the university. As a mentor you may be involved in identifying potential barriers and possible reasonable adjustments to overcome or remove those barriers for your student and will definitely be involved in the implementation of the adjustments that have been agreed as reasonable for your student.

Activity 11.2 Anticipatory reasonable adjustments

Take a walk round your organization and your workplace and identify what adjustments are already in place for disabled people or policies/processes/equipment that are inclusive of disabled people rather than excluding them. Also consider whether there are any you have in place specifically for students.

It is important to note that the university and placement providers also have an *anticipatory duty*. This means that the university and placement providers should have in place systems and processes for making reasonable adjustments in anticipation of having disabled students and do not wait until a disabled student arrives.

For example, universities will have in place a policy on assessment processes that will include provisions for adjustments to examination processes; for example, students with dyslexia may require extra time to complete an examination. Activity 11.2 requires you to consider adjustments that may already be in place where you work.

Adjustments/processes or equipment that you may have identified as already being in place might be:

- access ramps
- accessible toilets
- parking bays for disabled people
- loop systems for hearing aid users
- information booklets in large font or different-coloured paper
- taped handovers for people with visual impairments
- flashing phones/alarms for people with hearing impairments
- text phones
- computers.

We will come back to reasonable adjustments later in the chapter.

DISABILITY AND THE NMC

The NMC's prime function is to safeguard the public. It does this by setting the standards for education programmes, monitoring the quality of those programmes and giving guidance and advice to the professions.

The NMC do not bar anyone with a disability/ies from entering nursing programmes (this would be against the Disability Discrimination Act) but they do set the minimum entry criteria for nursing programmes which relate specifically to academic criteria. They also require both the education institution and their placement providers to ensure that they themselves meet the requirements of the Disability Discrimination Act (1995, 2005) which means that the education institution has to undertake the necessary checks to ensure applicants have 'the capability for safe and effective practice without supervision' (NMC, 2008). All applicants undergo a health check and if they have disclosed a disability then the student is offered advice and support through the university's occupational health and disability services. The university and placement providers also have a responsibility to ensure that their staff are aware of their role and responsibilities in relation to students with a disability.

Guidance for universities and placement providers are set out in the NMC's (2008) *Good Health and Good Character Guidance for Education Institutions* document, which is available on the NMC website. This is a useful guide to look at as it also has some scenarios related to disabled students which can help you understand how students can be supported.

The NMC also discuss the role of the mentor in relation to students with disabilities in their *Standards to Support Learning and Assessment in Practice* (NMC, 2008). Although rather brief it sets out the importance of promoting equality of opportunity and treating students with fairness, respect and understanding. It also highlights the importance of the university and practice working together to prepare staff for supporting students and preparing students for their practice placements.

THE IMPLICATIONS OF THE DDA FOR THE MENTOR

Put simply, you are legally required to comply with the DDA and professionally required to comply with the standards laid down by the NMC. However, you are not expected to find out about this by yourself; both your employer and the university have responsibilities.

Your employer should provide equality and diversity training that will encompass information on disabilities. This is usually a mandatory session that staff have to attend on a regular basis. Universities are required by the NMC to include information on supporting disabled students within its mentor preparation programmes and are also expected to work with practice partners to ensure mentors are prepared and supported for mentoring disabled students. All mentors are required by the NMC to update annually and these updates should also encompass information on mentoring disabled students.

Your responsibilities therefore are to:

- attend/complete statutory/mandatory training on equality and diversity
- ensure you update yourself as a mentor annually
- identify any gaps in your knowledge regarding you role in working with and supporting both students and colleagues who have a disability and seek to rectify those gaps
- seek guidance and support from the university or senior colleagues at work when you are unsure how to proceed if you are mentoring a student with a disability
- support students with a disability, treating them no less favourably than you would any other student
- implement reasonable adjustments to ensure that students are not discriminated against.

KEY POINT

Make sure you attend statutory/mandatory training as required on diversity and equality training and mentor updates annually.

DISCLOSURE

It is quite possible that you have worked with or mentored a disabled student but were completely unaware of their disability. This may be because it was a hidden impairment or disability and they had decided not to tell you about it. Often this is because a student feels able to manage their disability without any adjustments being required and so did not see the need to inform you. However, there are students who do not tell their mentor about their disability because their previous experiences of disclosing have resulted in less than positive attitudes by others either towards their disability or to disabled students in general.

Informing someone about a disability is called *disclosure*. Students have the right not to disclose their disability or to decide whom they wish to disclose to. If they restrict who is informed they are advised that this may limit the support that the university or practice can provide.

Under the DDA (1995, 2005) and SENDA (2001) the university and placement providers as public bodies are required to provide opportunities for students to disclose throughout their programme. This is not a one-off event and it is important that information for disabled students is widely available so that they are aware of their rights and the processes available to them to access support. At the very least, information will be provided in programme/course handbooks and on the university website.

WHAT ARE THE STEPS FOLLOWING DISCLOSURE?

Students may disclose their disability on their application form, at interview or at any point during the programme. When disclosed on the application form the university will usually contact the student and invite them to meet with a Disability Team Advisor to discuss the support that they will need whilst studying at the university. In the case of nursing students they will also need to discuss the support the student will require during their practice placements. If a student discloses after starting the programme they will be referred to the Disability Team at that point.

When the Disability Team Advisor meets with the student they will discuss with the student who will need to be informed about their disability/ies in order for reasonable adjustments to be put in place. The student will sign consent as to whom disclosure can be shared with, and if they limit who can be told they will be informed that this will affect the level of support that can be provided. In some cases the student may be happy to share details regarding the reasonable adjustments they require but not details of their impairment or disability.

The Disability Team Adviser will also be able to advise the student on the disability support funding available and how to apply for it. This money is to cover additional costs that may arise because of the student's disability and is not means tested. The funding allowances available are:

- specialist equipment allowance, e.g. computer, specialist furniture, electronic stethoscopes
- non-medical helper's allowance – to pay for a support worker, communication support worker or personal assistant
- general expenditure allowance
- travel allowance – to pay for travel expenses that are additional to those other students pay for (e.g. taxi fare rather than bus fare).

The student and the Disability Team Advisor will then draw up an agreement of the reasonable adjustments required; this may be called an Individual Support Plan or Agreement for Reasonable Adjustments. It is important to note that it can take time for the allowances to be applied for and agreed and so the specialist equipment to be acquired therefore the earlier the student meets with the Disability Support Team the better.

If the student has consented, a member of staff responsible for practice placements, and ideally a representative from practice, will meet with the student and the Disability Team Advisor to discuss the reasonable adjustments that the student will require whilst on practice placements and whether there are any difficulties with certain types of placement. Ideally

Case study 11.1 *Meeting competence standards*

1. A student with a hearing impairment is required to demonstrate competence in taking baseline observations. She achieves this on a ward placement by using an electronic monitor with a visual display to show blood pressure. There is no requirement in the competence standards that she has to specifically use a standard stethoscope.
2. A student with dyscalculia is allowed to use a calculator when calculating drug dosages.
3. A student who has been diagnosed with dyslexia uses a computer to write up the notes for patients in his care. This requires him to have some extra time in the working day to undertake this. There is no requirement in competence standards that he has to be able to write them with a pen nor that they have to be completed within a specified time frame.

the placements for the whole programme will be looked at to identify any that may pose significant challenges.

General factors to consider when considering each placement might be:
- distance from transport links
- accessibility at the actual placement
- noise levels
- light levels
- flexibility of work patterns.

It is important to note that the focus on making reasonable adjustments is on what needs to be put in place to enable the student to meet the competence standards of the programme. Competence standards themselves will not be changed but how the student is expected to perform and be assessed against these may need to be adjusted. Case study 11.1 gives an example.

THE MENTOR's RESPONSIBILITY IN RELATION TO DISCLOSURE

As a mentor you have a responsibility to create an environment in which all students feel comfortable to discuss confidential information with you. This includes enabling them to feel comfortable to disclose their disability to you and/or discuss the reasonable adjustments that they may require. At your first meeting with any student you should always ask them whether there are any reasonable adjustments that they require whilst on placement. This gives them the opportunity to disclose a disability if they have one and discuss reasonable adjustments required. In some cases a student may prefer to discuss reasonable adjustments without disclosing their actual disability. This is their right.

Since a student can disclose at any time on their programme you could be faced with a number of scenarios:

1. The student has disclosed at the university and reasonable adjustments have been agreed and the student:
   (a) Arranges to meet with you in advance or on the first day to discuss the reasonable adjustments they require.
   (b) Decides not to inform you until later in the placement when they feel comfortable with you or they wait until they run into difficulties related to their disability.
2. The student has not disclosed to the university – no reasonable adjustments are agreed and the student:
   (a) Discloses that they have a disability to you during their placement.
   (b) Does not disclose that they have a disability but you believe they may have one.

Let's look at these scenarios in turn.

Student discloses at the university and reasonable adjustments have been agreed in advance

The ideal situation is that the student will have visited you prior to the start of their placement so that the adjustments required can be discussed in advance. Depending on what adjustments are required and who the student has agreed this can be shared with, people who may be involved at the first meeting could be:

- The student
- The mentor and/or manager of the placement
- The student's personal tutor/the link lecturer
- The Disability Team Advisor from the university
- The person with responsibility for equality and diversity in your organization.

Student discloses at the university and reasonable adjustments have been agreed in advance but they do not inform you until later in the placement

As soon as a student discloses to you, the reasonable adjustments agreed have to be put in place.

Student discloses but doesn't have any reasonable adjustments agreed

Sometimes the student has chosen not to disclose to the university either because they believe they can manage any adjustments required without additional help or did not appreciate that they might require reasonable adjustments to be made when on placement until they got there. Consider Jenny's case in Case study 11.2.

Having regular meal breaks is a reasonable adjustment and a requirement by law; however, there are additional questions you may wish to ask such as:

- What happens if your diabetes becomes unstable?
- What are the signs we should be aware of?
- What actions should we take?
- If you should have a hypoglycaemic attack or become unwell is there anyone we should contact?
- Who else on this placement can I tell that you have diabetes?

If the student requests that no one else is to be informed about their diabetes you will need to discuss what information can be shared: for example, informing staff that your student requires regular meal breaks without giving the reason why. However, you will also need to point out that in restricting the information that can be shared should she have a hypoglycaemic episode this could have serious implications for her if you as her mentor were not around as staff may not recognize what is happening. The student may therefore decide that she will inform people on a need-to-know basis.

Case study 11.2

Jenny was diagnosed with diabetes when she was a child and has to inject herself with insulin twice a day. She manages her diabetes well and doesn't perceive herself as disabled, so has not contacted the disability support unit at the university. On her first day on placement Jenny informs her mentor that she has diabetes and therefore needs to have regular meal breaks.

Student has not disclosed to anyone but you believe they may have a disability/ies

A student may decide not to disclose their disability but it is either apparent to you because it can be seen; for example, the student wears a hearing aid or it may be that you suspect that they may have a hidden disability which has become apparent from their performance on the placement (e.g. dyslexia).

By asking all students whether they require any reasonable adjustments at the start of their placement you can pre-empt this. If they have a disability that is obvious then under the DDA reasonable adjustments must be put in place; however, this could be difficult if you do not know exactly what adjustments the student requires. If you find yourself in this position your first course of action should be to discuss with the student whether there are any reasonable adjustments that they may require on their placement. If the student is insistent that none are required it is important to record this in their practice assessment document. You should then contact the university to discuss this with the disability team whilst maintaining confidentiality about the student. They will be able to advise you on how you can best support the student during their placement.

If you believe a student may have a hidden disability based upon their performance or behaviour on the placement but they have not disclosed a disability nor requested reasonable adjustments this will require sensitive handling. Where you have concerns regarding any student's performance it is important to document any discussions you have with them in their practice assessment document and agree clear action plans. Contact the link lecturer or student's personal tutor and invite them to meet with you and the student to discuss your concerns.

KEY POINT

At the initial interview ask all students whether there are any reasonable adjustments they may require during their placement.

While on their placement it is quite possible that students may learn more about their disability/ies and may be involved in caring for people with the same or similar disabilities. This could be viewed positively by the student or create anxiety about their own disability. It is important to be sensitive to this and offer students the opportunity to discuss this experience with you.

Some students may need to attend support sessions during their placement such as study skills tuition or mentoring. It is important that they are allowed to attend these as these will be part of the reasonable adjustments identified for them. You will need to discuss with the Link Teacher whether this time counts as part of their clinical hours or whether an agreement has been made to enable the student to make-up any missed time in order to meet the NMC requirement that all students complete 2300 hours over a three-year programme.

DISCLOSURE AND CONFIDENTIALITY

If a student discloses to you, there are a number of issues to consider around confidentiality.

Under the Data Protection Act you may not disclose details about a person's disability without their consent. It is therefore important to discuss with the student whom they have already disclosed this to.

If this is the first time they have disclosed to anyone and they request that no one else is informed you will need to explain that whilst you will be able to make reasonable adjustments in the way that you support the student any adjustments that require specialist equipment or require actions by the organization you work for or by the university cannot be put in place. You should explain that by informing the disability support team at the university a more co-ordinated approach can be taken and will also allow the student to access specific funds through the disability student allowance, if needed, which can help provide specialist equipment, funding for a personal assistant or travel expenses.

If the student discloses to you and has an Individual Support Plan in place but does not wish anyone else to know about their disability then you should discuss how they want to share the Individual Support Plan with other colleagues they will be working with. They may request that you share this with colleagues on their behalf or decide they will share it with colleagues on a need-to-know basis. Again it is important that the student understands that limiting who knows can impact on the level of support provided.

It is also important to discuss with your student whether they wish to disclose their disability to the patients/clients they are caring for. Again this is their decision but they may seek your professional opinion in making this decision. Again the decision should be recorded.

THE STUDENT'S RESPONSIBILITY

The DDA clearly sets out the rights of people with disabilities. However, with rights come responsibilities and there are certain responsibilities that the student has in relation to their disability which include:

- To accept that if they do not disclose their disability to key staff then this will limit the support that can be provided.
- To be actively involved in identifying the reasonable adjustments they require and the development of their Individual Support Plan.
- To inform relevant staff where there are problems with implementing the agreed adjustments or they are insufficient to enable them to participate in the learning experiences.
- To access the Disability Team at the university and any other support networks that are available. This may also include the Disability Advisor at the placement if there is one in post.

The student is an expert on their disability and how it affects them and so it is imperative that their experience of what strategies and adjustments work for them are discussed and taken into account. No two students with the same disability will necessarily require the same adjustments.

REASONABLE ADJUSTMENTS FOR SPECIFIC IMPAIRMENTS OR DISABILITIES

This section looks briefly at the more common disabilities/impairments that students may require reasonable adjustments for.

BLOOD-BORNE INFECTIONS, HIV/HEPATITIS B AND C

Information about the student's condition will have been passed to the programme leader and placement manager so that they are placed where no exposure-prone procedures take place. There should therefore be no need for the student to tell their mentor about their diagnosis.

Should a student have an accident in placement, for example, a cut or a needlestick injury they should follow the normal accident reporting procedure, complete the placement and university incident/accident forms and ensure that they follow infection control procedures such as covering up cuts or wounds.

CHRONIC FATIGUE SYNDROME

Students may have difficulties with concentration, handling lots of tasks at once, stamina or memory. Examples of reasonable adjustments which students may find helpful include:

- adjustment to shift times and patterns
- regular breaks
- being allocated a smaller group of patients/clients to care for

- placements which do not require long travelling times
- use of notes/checklists.

DIABETES MELLITUS

Students are encouraged to inform their mentor about their condition and how they might behave before they have a hypoglycaemic episode and contact details for someone if they become suddenly ill. Students should discuss with you about wearing a MedicAlert identification system. A MedicAlert necklace may be worn but not a bracelet. Students should adhere to the university uniform policy.

Examples of reasonable adjustments which students may find helpful include:

- regular meal breaks
- time off to attend hospital/doctor appointments.

EPILEPSY

With epilepsy there may be unexpected relapses in the control of the condition, possibly due to the effects of longer days and the general stresses of coping with learning new skills and responsibilities in clinical areas. It is important to be aware of triggers previously not encountered. For example, where photosensitivity is a problem photographic angiography or radiographic departments may cause difficulties. Some students may experience concentration difficulties, side effects of medication and fatigue due to lack of sleep. A MedicAlert necklace may be worn but not a bracelet. Students must comply with the university policy.

It is important to agree with the student what action should be taken if they experience an aura, the actions that should be taken if they experience a seizure and how much recovery time they might need.

Reasonable adjustments are likely to focus around the avoidance of triggers. If the student knows the potential triggers for their seizures, they will need to discuss these with you so you can help them to identify/avoid the relevant departments/equipments where the triggers may be found.

HEARING IMPAIRMENT

Students with a hearing impairment may experience barriers to communication, such as noise levels, lighting, accents, verbal alerts and auditory alarms. It is important to discuss with the student their individual circumstances and the support they require.

Examples of reasonable adjustments which students may find helpful include:

- equipment for taking vital signs that have visual displays, e.g. blood pressure and pulse monitors
- amplified stethoscopes
- vibrating alerts to signal a monitor's alarm
- vibrating alerts for fire or emergency alarms
- ensuring you face the student when communicating with them if they lip read
- use of a British Sign Language interpreter
- text telephones
- amplified telephone
- placements that are smaller/quieter without too much background noise.

MENTAL HEALTH DIFFICULTIES

Mental health difficulties can fluctuate and therefore the student's support requirements may also fluctuate. At the initial interview discuss with the student what behaviour they may exhibit that would indicate they are becoming unwell. If a student appears to be unaware of a change in behaviour that indicates a relapse in their condition or mental distress which does not appear to be being managed well, please identify this with them and explore any coping strategies that they may have and how they can be implemented. Should this not be sufficient you should contact the link lecturer for additional advice.

Examples of reasonable adjustments which students may find helpful include:

- flexible work patterns to enable optimum performance
- modify workloads if required
- allow time off to attend hospital appointments.

SICKLE CELL/THALASSAEMIA

The main focus with sickle cell/thalassaemia is in ensuring your student maintains their health status. Ensure your student keeps themselves well hydrated and has their pain relief with them. Ask for a contact number should they experience a crisis.

Examples of reasonable adjustments which students may find helpful include:

- ensure appropriate breaks to reduce the risk of increased tiredness and help with concentration

- adjustments to shifts may be necessary
- student must be allowed to keep outpatient appointments as this is important to monitor their condition.

SPECIFIC LEARNING DIFFICULTIES

Specific learning difficulties such as dyslexia, dyspraxia, attention deficit hyperactivity disorder, or dyscalculia are recognized and covered as disabilities by disability legislation. Students with specific learning difficulties may have different support requirements outlined in their placement Individual Support Plan (see Box 11.2). Different aspects of placements may present different barriers to students with specific learning difficulties.

Mentors should discuss and identify with the student potential aspects of placements that may present barriers and discuss possible solutions/reasonable adjustments to remove barriers. This should be reviewed on a regular basis.

Examples of reasonable adjustments which students may find helpful include:

- regular opportunities to ask questions
- repeating instructions/allowing student to write instructions down
- recorded handovers they can listen to as needed
- providing examples of well-completed documentation
- access to a computer
- additional time to take notes/complete documentation
- lists of terms, abbreviations and common conditions
- use of a calculator
- use of coloured overlays.

VISUAL IMPAIRMENT

It is important that a student with a visual impairment has an orientation to the physical layout of the placement, preferably before the first day of the placement. Discuss with the student if the lighting levels are sufficient in the placement area for the student to be able to work night shifts, if the occasion arises. Individuals with a visual impairment can suffer night blindness in low light levels.

Examples of reasonable adjustments that students may find helpful include:

- handouts or information for students such as an induction pack; this should be provided in their preferred format (larger font, different coloured paper)

If the student is failing despite reasonable adjustments then you will need to develop an action plan and follow the guidance in Chapter 8 in this book. In the majority of cases all will go well and your student will achieve their competencies and pass their placement and you will have both learnt a lot from the experience which will be invaluable in supporting future students.

EVALUATING YOUR SUPPORT OF THE STUDENT WITH A DISABILITY

Once reasonable adjustments have been put in place, don't think that is it. It is very important to monitor their effectiveness on a regular basis throughout the placement to ensure they are continuing to meet the student's needs.

For example Jenny, who we looked at in Case study 11.2, may find that despite regular meal breaks, working long days is impacting on her blood sugar levels and so she requests to do a combination of early and late shifts in order to meet her practice hours. This would be a reasonable adjustment but may require a rethink of your off-duty to ensure that she continues to be supported through the placement.

At the end of the placement it is important that you evaluate how you and your workplace responded to the student's needs. The checklist in Box 11.3 offers possible questions you may wish to ask yourself. If you tick no for any you need to consider how you can improve on this area for the future.

Box 11.3 Checklist for evaluating a student placement that required reasonable adjustments

- Did the student make contact in advance of the placement?
- Did the student visit the placement before starting to discuss the reasonable adjustments they required?
- Did you discuss their Individual Support Plan prior to or at the start of the placement?
- Did you agree who (if anyone) could be informed of the student's disability/reasonable adjustments?
- Did you orientate the student to the placement on their first day?
- Did you meet with your student on a regular basis to review/monitor the effectiveness of any reasonable adjustments made?
- If any problems were encountered on the placement did you seek advice/support?

TOP TIPS

- Ask all students if they require reasonable adjustments.
- Always seek advice from the university if you are unsure how to best support a student with a disability.
- Never lower the standard of competence required just because a student has a disability.
- Seek regular feedback on whether reasonable adjustments are meeting the needs of the student.

RESOURCES

All universities will have a section of their website devoted to students with disabilities which you may find helpful. Some universities also have a separate area on their website for mentors which may also contain additional information or web links on disabilities.

References

Disability Discrimination Act (DDA) 1995. HMSO, London.

Disability Discrimination Act 2005. HMSO, London.

Nursing and Midwifery Council, 2008. Standards to Support Learning and Assessment in Practice: NMC standards for mentors, practice teachers and teachers. Nursing and Midwifery Council, London. Available from www.nmc-uk.org.

Special Educational Needs and Disability Act (SENDA) 2001. HMSO, London.

CHAPTER 12

MENTORING CHALLENGES

Chapter Aims

The purpose of this chapter is to explore the different challenges that you may encounter as a mentor. After reading this chapter you will be able to:
- Identify mentoring challenges in your clinical learning environment.
- Reflect on how you manage challenges.
- Identify practical measures to address challenges without compromising the assessment of learning.

INTRODUCTION

In the course of mentoring students you will experience a number of situations that may impact on the learning experience you aim to provide and on your perception of students. These situations may leave you feeling frustrated at times with your role as a mentor. This chapter endeavours to cover a variety of the situations that you may encounter, allowing you to assess your mentoring skills and offer practical solutions to help you support the student effectively.

MENTORING STUDENTS ON A SECOND ATTEMPT

One of the biggest challenges you will face as a mentor will be associated with the need to fail a student at the conclusion of a practice placement. We looked at the support for a failing student in Chapter 8. This section looks at failing a student at their final attempt at their practice assessment.

When a student submits their theory assignment there will be a delay before the results are officially released to the student. However, practice assessment is very different; the student will know the outcome immediately. If a student has failed an aspect of their practice assessment then they will know that you have failed them. It is likely that both of you will feel especially awkward about this, as you will have worked together over many weeks and no doubt built up a rapport. There may even be the added potential for conflict if there is disagreement about your assessment decision. The accuracy and reliability of feedback that you have provided throughout the placement will be especially valuable here. If a student has been prepared and supported for the likelihood of not achieving placement learning outcomes then the final decision will not come as a shock; however given that failing at a second attempt is likely to lead to discontinuation from the programme this is probably the most difficult situation you will face (see Case study 12.1).

Case study 12.1 *A link lecturer speaks of her experience of failing a student*

'I got a call from a mentor one Friday afternoon telling me that she had just failed a student who had taken the news very badly and had locked herself in an interview room. I rushed to the clinic and found the student sitting in the dark sobbing and crying. It became clear that the mentor had had misgivings about the student's competence during the previous eight weeks of the placement, but had felt unable to speak with the student as she didn't want to upset her. On the final day, the mentor had simply signed a number of outcomes as 'not achieved' and hoped that the student would understand. The student was devastated, she had no warning that she was likely to be failed and all trust in her mentor had gone. It was just a terrible situation, desperately trying to pick up the pieces of this student whose world had just collapsed. I wouldn't wish that on anyone.'

WHAT IS A SECOND ATTEMPT?

All university students are usually entitled to at least one further attempt of any assessment they have failed to pass. In this case a student is *referred* by the university which usually entitles a student to a second attempt at the learning outcomes they failed to achieve. The location, time and length of a practice placement to undertake the second attempt are decided upon by the university and dependent on the needs of the individual student. The student may not undertake their second attempt in the same placement as the first attempt as usually both mentor and student benefit from a fresh start. If a student were to request a second attempt in their first placement then this would be considered by the university, but only if the mentor and placement area were also in agreement.

THE MENTOR'S ROLE FOR A SECOND ATTEMPT

As students will usually be given a second attempt at any failed learning outcomes you may come across a student who did not pass on a previous placement and requires a second attempt with you. This could be quite challenging, as the student may enter the placement with low self-esteem or feeling very anxious and worried. Essentially, your role as a mentor will not alter and you will still be expected to provide a range of learning opportunities and provide a fair and accurate assessment. All the advice given in earlier chapters around the assessment process applies. To recap these are:

- undertake the initial interview as soon as possible in the first week.
- look at the mentor's comments from the placement where the student failed at the first attempt and at the comments in the ongoing achievement record.
- identify the learning outcomes to be achieved and agree a clear action plan with SMART objectives to help the student achieve those learning outcomes.
- meet regularly and give honest feedback on their progress.
- if the student is not meeting the required level of competence seek help from the university for you and the student as soon as possible.

Clear and consistent feedback is probably one of the most essential elements as the student will need to be informed of their progress and to be informed early on if they are not making the required progress. As the second attempt is a student's opportunity to demonstrate that they have developed and improved on the first attempt you should have a very clear benchmark to work from. The content and accuracy of the ongoing achievement record will be invaluable as you should be able to pick up from where the last mentor left off.

FIRST AND SECOND ATTEMPTS TOGETHER

In some circumstances students may be required to undertake their second attempt at failed learning outcomes at the same time as undertaking a new placement with new learning outcomes. This will usually happen when only a small number of learning outcomes are outstanding and it is not in the student's interest to restrict their progression. When you are mentoring a student who needs to undertake a second attempt on a practice assessment, remember you will only be assessing the student on the learning outcomes which they have not achieved during their first attempt. Students who are completing first attempts of one module and second attempts of another may have two practice assessment books and two sets of learning outcomes to be assessed. This means you will need to be very organized in your mentoring role to support this student. Remember however, that you should have the ongoing achievement record written by the mentor of the first attempt placement as a reference point. This should give you a good indicator as to what the student's areas for development and any issues and concerns are. Reflecting on the contents of the ongoing achievement record with the student will help the development of the action plans for the placement.

KEY POINT

Discuss the student's development /action plan with colleagues so they can support the student more effectively if there are times when you are not available for the student.

ASSESSING MULTIPLE LEARNING OUTCOMES

In those circumstances where you are being asked to assess the student on learning outcomes from both first and second attempts, your skills of planning for and facilitating learning will come to the fore. It is advisable to undertake an initial, midpoint and final interview for each set of learning outcomes. This will help distinguish what is required for each assessment and though a little more documentation is involved it will enable the student to focus on what needs to be done for each learning outcome. An ongoing achievement record should also be written after a second attempt, regardless of the outcome. Box 12.1 summarizes the terminology used by universities in the assessment process.

MAKING THE FINAL ASSESSMENT DECISION

The final assessment decision should never come as a surprise to the student. Throughout their placement with you, you will have given regular feedback on their progress and so they will know what the final outcome will be. As long as you have followed due process with documented evidence of a clear action plan with regular feedback, if the student has still been unable to achieve the required level of competence then your final decision has to be to fail the student. Always seek support from the

Box 12.1 Understanding university language

The language used by universities to indicate assessment processes may be confusing for mentors who are not used to the terminology. The following list includes some examples of such terms.

12-week rule	Nursing students have to pass all first year theory and practice assessments within 12 weeks of starting the branch programme in order to progress any further on the programme.
5-day rule	Submitting assessments within 5 working days after the deadline.
Appeal	Option available to a student if they do not agree with a decision made by assessment/mitigation boards but requires certain conditions to be met.
Applying for mitigation	The student submits evidence of extenuating circumstances which they believed affected their academic performance and therefore the outcome of the assessment.
Deferred	Results have yet to be released until additional requirements are submitted for the assessment.
Extension request	Option available to the student to apply for an extension to the submission date of the assessment – usually no more than 10 working days.
Fitness to practice/ disciplinary hearing	A panel of academic staff and practice representative(s) who consider an allegation of a breach or breaches against university regulations or the Student Code of Conduct which bring into question a student's fitness to practice.
Mitigation	Defined as the taking into account of any circumstances which were not within the foresight and control of the student and which the university believes might adversely affect the academic performance of a student.
Ratified results	Final results released by the university assessment board.
Referred	Did not pass first attempt.
Second first attempt	The student is permitted to undertake another first attempt of the practice placement due to accepted mitigating circumstances or due process not being followed.

university in this situation. This will be a difficult interview to undertake and so having a link lecturer sitting in on the final assessment will provide support to you and the student. Afterwards you may find it helpful to discuss the whole process with the link lecturer to assure yourself that you did all that was required and identify what you have learnt from this process.

THE WORK–LIFE BALANCE

The student population is changing and in many parts of the country the majority of students starting preregistration nursing courses are aged over 25. Many students will have non-traditional qualifications such as NVQ, Access in Healthcare, or may not have been in education for some time. Not all will have worked in healthcare before. We are also seeing more students coming into nurse education after starting a family or having decided on a significant career change.

All of the above can lead to challenges as the student is faced with juggling the demands of family, friends, shifts and coursework commitments. The student may request changes to shifts or decline to do certain shift patterns during their practice experience. While you may feel very tempted to allow students to request a specific rota out of kindness, this can result in the student not being on duty with you therefore limiting your opportunity to assess their performance.

As difficult as it may be, reinforcing the need for the student to be on duty with you for at least 40% of the time that they are delivering patient care and undertaking a variety of shifts is necessary. The NMC requires students to participate in the full range of care across 24 hours, including weekends and night duty and students can feel frustrated by what they may perceive as strict rules and regulations. It's a good idea to confirm with the university the expectations they have regarding students' working patterns and ensure these policies are maintained in your practice area.

Consistency is as important between placements as it is between mentors and this is not easy to achieve. Attending education meetings at organization and local level and discussing such issues is an ideal way to share good practice and agree approaches to enhance continuity. Of course there will be times that you exercise your professional judgement and allow the student to choose or swap shifts but this must not be at the expense of their learning needs. Students must complete a minimum

Case study 12.2 *A mentor's experience of planning an off-duty*

'A few years ago I was sitting with my student at the end of the initial interview and we were completing her off duty for the month. I knew that the student needed to do two weekends and one week of nights and I wanted her to do these with myself. The student explained she had small children and wanted to be at home at the weekends, she said her previous placements had always let her work more early shifts and gave her weekends off. Because the placement was 8 weeks long we eventually came to the agreement she would do the weekends and nights during the fifth and sixth weeks to allow her time to arrange childcare. It wasn't an easy conversation, I felt like I was being the bad guy and our relationship didn't get off to the best start. I found out later that the other ward had not given her weekends off at all; she was just testing me to see if I would give in. Now our Trust just makes it clear to all students that we follow the university policy for student placement and we don't have any more problems.'

number of hours across the 24-hour period and failure to achieve this is not in keeping with course requirements or professional in behaviour. Persistent and consistent changes to off-duty or refusal to do certain shifts can be assessed against the relevant learning outcome and involvement of the academic link is advisable. See Case study 12.2.

KEY POINT

Use the initial interview to establish with the student any special circumstances the student may have that could prevent them undertaking their designated off duty. Seek advice from the university if the student will be unable to commit to the placement.

BEREAVEMENTS

There could be a time when you are informed by the student that a relative or friend has died and they would like time off to grieve and travel to the funeral. In these situations the student could need more time off than they initially requested. Leave from the course, including from placement, on compassionate grounds can only be authorized by the university.

As a mentor your role is to support the student to follow the correct reporting procedures, as well as offer the student an empathetic ear.

There may be times when the student does not wish to take time off from the placement or programme, believing that studying will provide a distraction and a way to cope with the loss. In these instances it is advisable to liaise with the academic link as additional support can be put in place for the student, this may be via occupational health or extra meetings with the student and yourself. Either way, the assessment process must be followed and your empathy for the student must not impact on the quality of your assessment. The academic link will also be available to support you and the student if you've identified poor performance.

FINANCE AND INCOME

Financial hardship is a reality for many students. Some students may find themselves in significant debt and for obvious reasons this may impact on their ability to learn on placement. Students who are concerned about paying bills will not be in the best frame of mind to take advantage of the learning experiences on a placement. Under these circumstances it is not uncommon to discover that students are undertaking paid work as bank or agency care assistants, which may lead to increased tiredness, reduced concentration and poor performance.

If a student discloses financial difficulties to you as a mentor this must not cloud the assessment process or decision. You can suggest that your student could do one of the following:

- access the students' union for advice and support
- meet with their personal tutor to discuss the impact of the financial hardship on their studies and the options available
- contact Citizens Advice Bureau or the National DebtLine.

If you suspect the student of working extensive hours on bank, agency or other paid employment but do not have the evidence you are advised to assess the student on the behaviour which is causing concern. For example, if the student is witnessed to fall asleep or found asleep whilst on duty you should do the following:

- ensure a minimum of two staff have observed the student to be asleep and witness statements are prepared
- meet with the student to discuss the behaviour; do not get into a heated 'he said, she said' discussion as this is unproductive; highlight which

learning outcome the lack of professionalism is being assessed against and how this incident will be monitored
- record the incident in the student's practice assessment document
- make an assessment of the student's alertness and liaise with the student's placement office if you decide the student should go home to sleep or rest and return to duty when fit to come back.

If you have been informed by colleagues from another department that your student was on duty the night before and they are now on placement during the day, immediate action needs to be taken to protect patients and the student. It is likely you will be sending the student home to sleep/rest until fit to return. You are advised to do the following:
- obtain statements from staff confirming the paid duties of the student
- meet with the student to discuss the allegation of poor professional conduct and breach of the student code of conduct. It is also helpful to establish their understanding of the impact of their actions
- contact the education lead in your organization (e.g. clinical placement facilitator, practice educator) and the link lecturer to inform them of the incident and agree a way forward
- liaise with the student's placement office to inform them of the outcome
- document the discussion and outcome in the student's practice assessment book.

PROFESSIONAL CONDUCT

As part of your assessment of a student's competence you are being asked to assess their professionalism. However, this can be complicated by our personal and professional view of acceptable standards and expectations. It is important to communicate and inform students of what your expectations and standards are as well as act in the manner required of the students.

Explaining to students and role modelling how you would like them to behave is very important. Do not assume that the students are aware of what is or is not considered professional in your clinical area, this is what they are there to learn. It can be difficult at times to articulate what we mean by 'behave professionally' and 'just watch me' might not be enough.

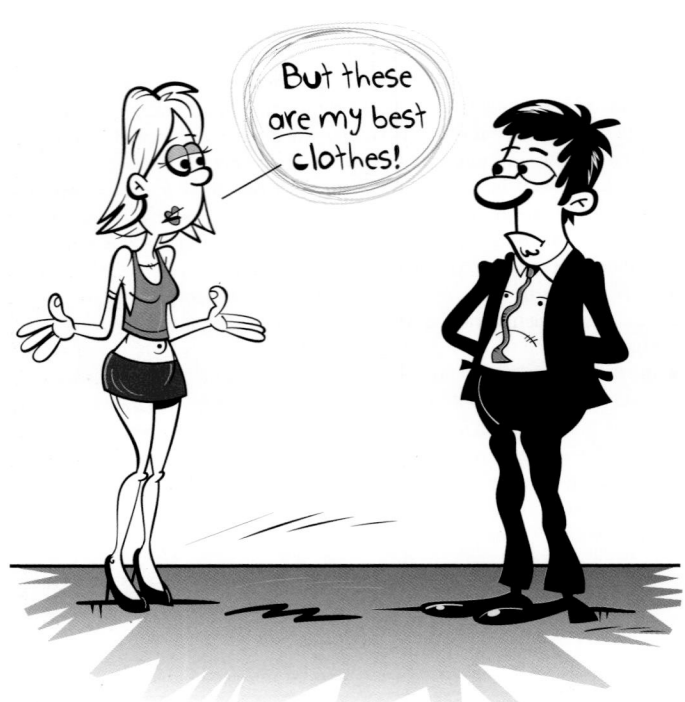

Aspects of professional behaviour that are expected:
- adherence to uniform policy
- punctuality
- informing you if they will be late/off sick
- demonstrating interest and motivation
- communicating with staff and patients in an appropriate manner
- taking responsibility for their own learning.

It is likely that you will think of more.

If your student is behaving in a manner which is less than professional try to avoid the parental approach of 'stop that', 'don't do that' as this can be demeaning. Instead, try to explain the reasons for your concerns and try to engage the student in deciding on an alternative approach that they will be comfortable with. See Case study 12.3.

Case study 12.3 *A student shares his experience of a patient visit*

'I was on my first community placement and we were going to assess this patient my mentor knew well. I was worried that I would not be able to remember everything that was said so when my mentor was talking to the woman I was making notes of her answers. My mentor noticed and gave me an odd look which made me feel uncomfortable. I wasn't sure what to do, so I stopped writing. Afterwards in the car my mentor asked me what I was doing making notes in front of the patient and that I shouldn't have done that because it was rude and unprofessional and I should have been listening to what was being said. I explained I was struggling to remember everything and didn't think it was that bad. My mentor told me I should have explained to the patient why I wanted to take notes and asked permission before doing anything. She explained that this patient can feel very vulnerable and paranoid if notes are taken about them, and it's best to listen and pay full attention rather than write notes. I realized that I have to ensure that I consider how my patient feels, not just do something because I feel like it.'

The following are some things which you can try with your students.
- Using positive statements which incorporate an explanation can illustrate what we do and why.
  - Try 'I would like you to be on time for duty so you can participate in handover' instead of 'you keep missing handover because you're late'
  - Try 'The Patients' Charter tells us that our clients/service users/patients/family/carers like to see staff wearing ID badges to help in recognizing different people' instead of 'Where's your ID badge?'
- Encourage reflection on behaviour and problem solving using questions such as:
  - How have you seen other staff approach X?
  - How do you think X might respond if you were to do. . . . . .?
- Use role play to try out unfamiliar situations. This is a good way to practise how to conduct oneself professionally.

Focusing on the behaviours rather than the presenting attitude will mean you can give concrete examples of what is or is not acceptable, this also limits the 'yes you are', 'no I'm not' discussion.

SICKNESS AND ABSENTEEISM

There will be times when your student calls in sick or calls to say their childcare arrangements have failed and so are unable to attend placement. Life happens; these moments can and do happen to everyone. The challenge and problems occur when the absenteeism (regardless of reason) is persistent and extended. Long periods of absence reduce the amount of time you can spend with the student to assess them thoroughly. It also means the student will struggle to demonstrate evidence of their learning.

It is important that the university placements office is informed of all absences regardless of the reason on the day the student is absent. This way a record is immediately kept but also the amount of absence can be tracked. If there has been no contact from the student to inform you of the reason they are absent letting the placements office know means they can attempt to make contact with the student to find out what has happened and ask them to call you. When the student returns to placement discuss why informing you that they will be absent is important and ensure that their timesheet is updated showing the time missed.

KEY POINT

Students must complete 2300 hours in practice and 2300 hours of theory in order to register with the NMC. If they miss time in practice they won't be able to register at the end of their programme.

If the student has been absent for extended periods or has been taking lots of odd days off and it feels like the student is not around at all, consider the following actions:

- review and double check the off duty – does it clearly state the shift the student did not attend and what type of absence it was? If there are gaps liaise with the staff who were on duty those days to confirm attendance or absence.
- inform the student's placement office of all the absences – if you email the information you can copy in the academic link or education lead so they are kept up-to-date.
- arrange to meet the student with the link lecturer on their return to placement to discuss the absence(s).
- if due to the extensive absences you cannot make a fair and just assessment of the student's competence you must inform the link lecturer as soon as possible and document this in the student's practice assessment book.

With the evidence of persistent absence the personal tutor or programme leader can use this to explore with the student their ability to meet the course requirements and identify any mitigating circumstances. If the student is not demonstrating an improvement in their time keeping and professionalism there could be a case for disciplinary action. Key to either scenario is the evidence in timesheets, practice assessment book and information provided to the placements office.

> **KEY POINT**
>
> Absenteeism that is not recorded officially with the university will remain hidden from future employers. Students with poor attendance records cannot be identified unless the university is informed of absenteeism by mentors.

INCIDENTS/ACCIDENTS

Occasionally, unfortunate accidents or incidents do occur and students may be involved themselves or are a witness to an incident or accident. For any accident or incident the procedures you follow for the student will not be that different from what you would do if it were a member of staff. Complete both the reporting form used by your organization and the university one (if they have one). A debrief is essential and so too is letting the academic link know so that they too can offer their support.

If the student requires medical intervention and is sent home sick the student's placements office should also be informed. When a student has been injured and required medical intervention, they should be seen by their GP and/or the university occupational health team to make an assessment and decision as to their fitness to return to placement. In some cases it may be helpful to have a three-way meeting with the student, academic link and mentor to reflect on the incident to gain a greater insight into what happened and to support the student if they are feeling overwhelmed by the experience.

PREGNANCY

You may find that you are required to mentor a student who is pregnant during their practice placement. When this happens the student will be required to meet with their lecturer to discuss and agree a pregnancy plan; this will include informing the placements office. Occasionally, some students do not wish to disclose their pregnancy for fear it will impact on their bursary and will slow their progression on the course. Pre-registration students are now entitled to continue to receive bursary payments if they take maternity leave during their programme and students are normally required to commence maternity leave from week 34 of their pregnancy.

The student will need a pregnancy risk assessment undertaken as soon as you are aware they are pregnant; this could be the first day of placement (if notified in advance) or at any point in the placement period depending on when the student finds out and/or informs you. In completing the risk assessment you will need to consider what limitations to the student's activities may be required and the impact on the student's ability to achieve their learning outcomes. If you feel the student will not be able to undertake a suitable range of practice experiences to meet the learning outcomes contact the link lecturer and/or trust education lead immediately. A decision can then be made as to the suitability of another practice area or whether the student may be required to commence their maternity leave forthwith. See Case study 12.4.

Case study 12.4 *A student speaks of her experience of being pregnant during a clinical placement*

In my third year I fell pregnant and started a placement in a really busy A&E department. On my first day my mentor said that when mobile X-rays were done in the department I should stand well back behind a screen. I didn't think it would be a problem but then it seemed every 20 minutes someone would need an X-ray and I would have to stop what I was doing and move behind this screen. In the end it just wasn't practical to stay there; I was just missing out on so many experiences. I was moved to a cardiology ward and the problem was solved.

If a pregnant student's health changes at any point after the risk assessment was completed and she can no longer engage in some learning opportunities it will be appropriate to redo the risk assessment. Once a student reaches 34 weeks in pregnancy a confirmation from the GP or midwife that the student is fit and well to remain in fulltime education is required. If the student is unable to produce this confirmation, maternity leave will begin immediately regardless of whether they are on placement or in a theory part of the course.

MOTIVATING STUDENTS

A significant part of the mentoring role is to motivate and encourage students; this may not always be easy because students have different learning styles and what works with one student may not motivate another. A student who feels encouraged and motivated will tell you they feel supported and that their mentor is interested in them and their development. Students who are not motivated during a practice placement can be especially challenging. It may be difficult to engage them in placement experiences and they may seem bored or disinterested. A student who is not motivated is unlikely to be learning, so it is important that you discover what the problem is and try to re-motivate them as quickly as possible. Some of the following may help to keep you and your students motivated:

- make students feel welcome in your unit/ward
- give constructive feedback regularly
- praise the student when they achieve something or do well
- make time at the beginning of the shift to ask the student what they wish to learn during the day and ask how you can help them with this
- set realistic goals with the student and stick to the plan
- regularly point out the connection between what the student is doing and their learning outcomes
- if the student does do something incorrectly or unprofessionally address it immediately
- be enthusiastic about your work and avoid being negative about colleagues in the presence of students
- keep your end of the bargain; if you said you will meet the student on Friday to review their learning that week then don't break this promise. Now undertake Activity 12.1.

Activity 12.1

Reflect on the last time you were mentoring or supporting a student.
  What did you do or say that you know helped this student perform?
  Was there anything that you felt you could have done differently?
  What have you learned from this experience that you can use to
improve your next mentoring experience?

STUDENT COMPLAINTS

As a mentor a student may approach you with concerns about inappropriate or below standard care they have observed or about how someone has treated them. This can be very challenging if a colleague or friend is the person identified and your instinct may be to defend them and disbelieve the student.

First, establish exactly what has happened from the student's perspective, what they saw, what was said. This will give you the opportunity to ask clarifying questions and time to reflect on the incident. Taking the time to understand what has happened can give you an insight into what is driving the complaint.

You will need to be very sensitive in the way you handle your initial investigation into the concern the student is reporting. There will be a number of factors that you should investigate initially.

- Has the student genuinely witnessed poor practice or have they witnessed an intervention that has been poorly explained and therefore they do not fully understand what they observed?
- Is there a personality clash between the student and a member of staff? Has there been any attempt to resolve the conflict?
- Has there been a misunderstanding that has been blown out of proportion?

These questions are not to belittle the student's experience, it is simply about trying to understand what has happened and ensure no misconceptions have arisen. The student may not feel empowered or confident to do more than tell you what has happened, however, you should remind them of the options available to them. These options could include:

- having a three-way meeting with the manager or academic link
- having a three-way meeting with the person with whom there is conflict
- putting the complaint in writing.

Reminding the student of their options allows them to make a decision as to what they want to do next. It may be appropriate to give the student some time to consider these.

In some circumstances it may be appropriate for a student to disclose their concerns confidentially and they should feel supported in doing this. You should therefore be aware of what mechanisms are in place in your practice area to ensure concerns can be raised privately, and how such concerns are dealt with. See Case study 12.5 and then undertake Activity 12.2.

Case study 12.5 Resolving conflict

An argument between a student and member of staff resulted in complaints and counter complaints being made about each other. The manager decided to let the student leave 30 minutes early from the shift to reflect on what had happened and hold a three-way meeting the next day. The next day everyone was much calmer. It was clear a misunderstanding had occurred, leading to the argument and was resolved amicably. The complaints were withdrawn and apologies accepted. During the meeting the manager took the opportunity to remind the student and staff about professional conduct and fed back to them how they were to discuss, negotiate and listen to each other following a period of reflection. In this example leaving the action till the next day allowed a quicker resolution.

Activity 12.2

Take some time now to investigate and reflect on the policies within your practice area related to raising concerns.

What are the students' raising concerns or whistle blowing procedures for your area?

What is the role of the mentor in such circumstances?

Always remain open to the possibility that the student might change their mind, from not wishing to pursue the complaint formally at all to deciding to do so after a time period has lapsed or at the end of a placement. Complaints about poor patient care may need a slightly different approach if what the student is describing are actions which breach a duty of care and you cannot wait for the student to decide what to do next. Discretion may be needed to investigate the issue to obtain all the facts.

The focus so far has been on the student making a complaint about something that does not directly involve you as a mentor. However, it might happen that the student does complain to the manager or link lecturer about your behaviour, actions or lack of action. The less experienced or confident a student is at dealing with conflict the more emotive the complaint may be in its content. This could lead to heated and difficult conversations without effective mediation. The most common cause is around the assessment process. Not following the process of the assessment can be distressing for the student and affect their faith in you as a mentor. They will be justified in complaining if the initial interview has not been completed in the first week or you regularly do not keep to arrangements to meet without explanation.

Any intervention from the link lecturer should mirror what you would do with your student if they came to you with a complaint. The aim is not to apportion blame, rather to establish an understanding of events and agree a way forward. See this as an opportunity to seek advice and have questions answered to enable you to undertake your role more effectively.

MANAGING A CROSSOVER OF STUDENT PLACEMENTS

At times, due to the nature and timing of placements across three years there could be a crossover of students in your placement. This can add to the number of people around, in some cases there could be more staff and students than patients! This may even result in a sense of competition amongst students for the best learning opportunities. It can also mean that some mentors may not have a break from assessing students if you have only a few 'live' mentors at the time. Preparation and planning for learning in these circumstances is essential and there are some things you can do to manage the crossover successfully.

- Ask the established student to orientate and induct the new student to the clinical area, the unit/hospital and staff.
- Ask the established student and new student to work together looking at a specific clinical issue encountered in that placement area, jointly prepare a presentation on the topic and then present it to the team at an agreed handover.
- Ask the established student to prepare detailed handover notes of the current patients, introduce and handover all the patients to the new student.
- Arrange for the new student to meet other professionals in the team during the crossover period.
- Consider spoke placements where some of the students can go for short periods, e.g. theatres during a surgical placement.
- Have a timetable of activities mapped out for the new student during the crossover.
- Have the off duty completed for the crossover period in advance so you can arrange for the students to be on shift with their mentor yet not all on the same shift at the same time. Undertake Activity 12.3.

KEY POINT

Asking the established student to be involved in orientating new students is an opportunity to assess the student's organization, planning, communication, leadership and team working skills.

Activity 12.3 Motivating students

Have a think about the learning opportunities in your placement area that could be utilized more effectively during the crossover? Make some brief notes now about how students could work together during these crossover periods.

REFUSING CARE FROM STUDENTS

More often than not patients, service users, carers and families do not object to students being present as an observer or participant in their care. Occasionally, patients will decline for students to be present or you might exercise your professional judgement and exclude the student. This can be frustrating for both the student and mentor. The challenge is helping students learn about the assessment and interventions you would be performing, understand why somebody might say 'no' and how decisions are made to exclude students from participating in care.

Here are a few suggestions of what you can do with your student on those occasions when they cannot participate in the care delivery process.

- Ask the student to review the patient's notes to look for indicators of why the patient may decline a student presence.
- Ask the student to review the patient's notes and care plans and identify where this specific assessment or intervention fits into the overall care.
- Ask the student to research the evidence base and organization's policies for the assessment or intervention you will be using – the student could do a presentation to you afterwards.
- Ask the student to engage in an activity which supports the intervention: e.g. preparation of the trolley and equipment ready for a wound dressing; calculating the drug dosage of an injection.
- Role play the assessment or intervention to be performed and encourage reflection in action to highlight how personal space could be invaded, how exposing it can feel and how impersonal the intervention may be.

Using activities such as this allow the student to learn about the specific assessment or intervention, participate to a point and not feel wholly excluded yet also help them understand the patient experience. By allocating the student a learning activity for the time you are with the patient, you have planned a learning experience and are indirectly supervising and supporting them. This can alleviate feelings of frustration associated with being excluded.

INVOLVING OTHER SERVICES/TEAMS

Having the support of others in the mentoring of students can relieve some of the anxiety of what to do with your student when you are not around as well as provide emotional and practical support if the student is not performing as well as you would hope. It can be very easy to suggest professionals and services a student should learn about through meeting or visiting without considering the other person's view of their role in the learning process.

Encouraging the involvement of some may require a different approach if they are not as proactive with student learning as you. One approach to indirectly encourage the involvement of other professionals or teams in student learning is preparation of the student who is going to meet them. This could involve the student preparing an updated summary of a patient's care that the professional is involved with and handing over this summary as well as finding out about how that professional provides care and support to the patient. Another alternative could be having information in the placement's information pack about the different roles and what can be learnt from each professional in the team which the student reads and then agrees what further questions to ask the professional that the information does not answer. Having worksheets for students to complete can help structure the learning experience as well as provide evidence towards their learning.

If it is possible, agree with the other professionals a fortnightly or monthly time slot when students could meet with them to find out about their role. This would be fixed in time and place and the other professionals would not be overwhelmed by lots of calls from students and you would be able to prearrange for the student to attend.

To help students engage with members of the multidisciplinary team you may like to develop worksheets that highlight the learning opportunities available (Box 12.2). The student will benefit from having a focused approach to the learning event, and the staff member they work with will be prepared to talk about specific aspects of their role and engage the student with the care they deliver where appropriate.

Box 12.2 Worksheet – learning about the different members of the MDT

Name of professional . . . .
Date & time of meeting with professional . . . .
Contact details for this professional . . . .

What are this professional's roles and responsibilities?

_____

_____

_____

How does this role differ from a nurse's role?

_____

_____

_____

When and how would you refer a client to this professional?

_____

_____

_____

MENTORING IN DIFFERENT TYPES OF PLACEMENT AREAS

Individual clinical areas will bring unique challenges to the mentoring and learning experience. These are generated by the nature of the service delivered. This could be the types of health problems treated, the health status of the patient group or the specialized nursing care delivered. There will always be some types of nursing and nursing care which preclude the involvement of students to a greater or lesser degree. However, there will always be similarities between professionals regardless of the setting. Commonly heard by students is 'you can learn that on your next ward placement' or 'you'll do plenty of that when you're in the community' and this is regardless of what pathway of nurse education the student is following.

COMMUNITY PLACEMENTS

Community services provide opportunities for students to learn how acute care and long-term care is provided in an alternative to the hospital environment. Community teams can be made up of different specialist nurses, usually of a senior grade with extensive work experiences. Many community teams operate Monday to Friday 9 am to 5 pm; however, there will be some that provide services 7 days a week, 365 days a year.

In community services when students are allocated a mentor they generally find themselves spending more time with this mentor compared to a mentor on a ward placement. This happens as a result of travelling to and from patient's homes, attending meetings together and students are less likely to engage in clinical duties by themselves or be indirectly supervised by their mentor. This perceived or actual experience of spending more time with the mentor can be stressful for the student as well as the mentor. The student may feel as though they are constantly being watched or not being allowed to have any independence. The mentor may feel the additional responsibilities of having a student an added stressor and a sense of not being able to have a break. For both, these feelings and perceptions may increase if the student is underperforming.

Below are some practical tips to help you mentor students successfully and manage the challenges of working in community settings, many of which you probably already do.

- Encourage the student to use a diary (but ensure patient/client confidentiality is not being broken).
- Provide a timetable of the week indicating the established meetings the student must attend, e.g. referral meetings, case conferences, student drop-ins and when home visits take place.
- Book into your diary when you will conduct the initial, midpoint and final interview and any other regular supervision meetings you will have – the student can then put these in their diary.
- Make a note of any study days the student has during the placement and if possible use these days to have your own supervision or see patients who would rather not see students.
- Allocate the students two to three patients whom they will get to know and learn how care is provided for these patients - this way the majority of your caseload is not overwhelmed by unfamiliar people whom they may only see once or twice.
- Ask the student to telephone patients whom you are planning they meet and work with, in advance of the first visit to introduce themselves.
- On days when the student is not participating in care for their allocated clients they can use this time to visit other services or meet with different professionals in the team.

One dilemma faced by mentors in community settings is whether they should let students do home visits by themselves. The NMC is very clear that any nurse or midwife who delegates duties to a junior member of staff including students remains accountable for those actions and the care delivered in their absence if allocated. It is advisable to double check if the university has a lone working policy specifically relating to students to guide you in making the decision to delegate unsupervised duties.

INPATIENT PLACEMENTS

In inpatient settings it is not unusual to have a greater capacity for students compared to community settings. Unlike many community services, inpatients wards could have an allocation of as many as six to eight students at any one time from any year of the programme. This may vary in specialist wards where only third-year students have placements. It also means that mentors could be supporting and assessing students on a more frequent basis adding to the stress of these additional responsibilities.

Listed below are some practical strategies to help manage the learning experience on an inpatient ward, again you might find you already do some of these.

- Have a rolling list of 'live' mentors so that responsibilities are shared.
- Arrange the off-duty so students are spread across the shifts but still with their mentors a minimum of 40% of the time whilst they deliver patient care.
- Allocate two to three patients to each student whom they will get to know and learn how care is provided for these patients.
- Agree two to three projects that the students can work together on during the course of their placements which they can have allocated time off the ward to research and prepare and present at an agreed handover.
- Encourage students to meet other professionals in the team or other services together.
- Encourage students to attend drop-in or support surgeries if run by the link lecturer.

For some of these practical solutions you will notice there are similarities between the community and inpatient settings. This is because the challenges faced are often the same, the only difference is the setting in which it takes place. This is not to discredit individual experiences rather illustrate where the common ground exists in mentoring.

WHERE TO FIND HELP

Whatever the challenge there are a range of resources available to help you. Always seek help if you are unsure, do not struggle on your own. Seeking help is not admission of failure, rather it is the professional thing to do when faced with an event about which you have limited knowledge or experience. Resources available to you are:

- other mentors
- link lecturer
- clinical placement facilitator
- practice educator/lecturer practitioner
- university website/placement website.

 TOP TIPS

- Make sure you have copies of the university policies relevant to students on practice placements.
- Find time to reflect on the way you handle any challenges with a student and how you might handle a similar situation next time.
- Share ideas for managing the student learning experience with colleagues on other placements.
- Always seek advice from the university if you are unsure how to respond to any situation involving a student.

CHAPTER 13

USING SIMULATED LEARNING

Chapter Aims

The purpose of this chapter is to gain insight into how simulation can be used in pre-registration nurse education. After reading this chapter you will be able to:

- Identify the key elements of simulated learning environments/simulation.
- Evaluate strengths and weaknesses of your own teaching style in relation to facilitating simulation.
- Plan effectively for a simulation session.
- Plan effectively for debriefing following simulation.

WHAT IS SIMULATED LEARNING?

Currently in all aspects of healthcare there is renewed focus on patient safety and quality indicators. Simulation-based training can help practitioners at all levels to reduce risk and improve the safety and quality of patient care. It is, however, most widely used in pre-registration programmes. You may feel this is only relevant to lecturers in the university but as this chapter will show simulation can be used and indeed is frequently used by mentors in practice. There is also increasing involvement of mentors in university simulation centres with the NMC seeing this as best practice.

First, don't be daunted. Simulation is simply another tool in your repertoire of teaching and learning skills and although it may include technologically advanced tools, it doesn't have to. The simulation process 'allows interactive, and at times immersive, activity by recreating all or part of a clinical experience without exposing patients to the associated risks' (Maran and Glavin, 2003 p. 22).

Students are required to respond to situations as they would in the clinical environment usually in real time, applying and integrating knowledge skills and critical thinking. Debriefing and feedback on performance is crucial to the process to ensure that learning is accompanied by assessment (usually informal) and reinforcement of good practice. Participants are active rather than passive receivers of information. This 'learning by doing' approach to learning is one that suits many nursing students.

WHY USE SIMULATION

Simulation is used in many disciplines, particularly when the reality may be dangerous, events are rare or errors are costly in human and/or financial terms. Obvious examples are the aviation industry, where sophisticated flight simulators are mandatory in the training of pilots to maintain their skills, the military and the nuclear power industry. Although the use of simulation and simulators has a relatively long history in medical and nursing education, it is only relatively recently that it has been recognized by the NMC as an essential component of nursing and midwifery programmes.

USING SIMULATION IN NURSE EDUCATION

Students on nursing programmes need to learn practical clinical skills in order to become competent. Some of these psychomotor skills are technically advanced; in the wider context of patient care many involve high levels of cognition, critical thinking and communication skills. It would appear that the acquisition and development of competence in these skills is becoming more challenging as the complexity of healthcare increases and the context changes. As modes of healthcare delivery change there may be less and less opportunities for students to experience certain aspects of care or practise specific skills during their placements. Students gain experience in a variety of settings other than acute care. Whilst this is entirely appropriate, it means that students' exposure to the hospital environment, where many clinical skills were traditionally honed, is reduced. Even in the hospital setting changing practices, for example, the increase in day case surgery, mean that students may not have the opportunity to practise certain skills, such as suture removal and injection techniques, as they once did. Mentors have many competing demands upon their time, whilst the NMC code of conduct requires all qualified nurses to support students, the needs of patients will by necessity take priority.

Against this background of an increasing patient safety and risk management agenda and reduced availability of clinical placements, the interest in and demand for simulation-based training has increased. Simulation is being recognized as a way of offering the opportunity to train multiprofessional groups of staff for real patient situations in a realistic context in a way that is risk free for patients and, if correctly facilitated, risk free for staff. Through simulation-based teaching, students are provided with the opportunity to rehearse skills, procedures and events not often used. They are also provided an opportunity to refine and develop skills used on a more frequent basis but which can not be rehearsed and practiced in the real environment for practical and/or ethical reasons.

SIMULATION IN CLINICAL PRACTICE

In recent years many healthcare organizations have invested in sophisticated manikins and other equipment in order to provide simulation-based training to staff, which you may have used. The NMC has agreed that pre-registration nursing students can spend up to 300 hours of their 2300 hours of practice time in simulated environment but recommends that mentors should be involved.

PROVISION OF SIMULATED LEARNING

There are many ways to provide simulation-based training. Sometimes simulation will involve highly sophisticated manikins, at other times it may involve actors or a mixture of both. Simulated learning can also take place in a virtual environment in the form of interactive computer-based learning packages. The key to all of these approaches is immersion. The scenario or patient situation created must be as realistic as possible in order that the participant becomes immersed in it and reacts and responds as if it were real. Simulation most often takes place in a university-based setting where students and practitioners come together to provide this experience with the support of the students' lecturers. Whilst these facilities are often well equipped and provide access to staff who are experienced in simulation, it requires a high level of planning and co-ordination to get everyone in the same place at the same time.

Increasingly, simulation is taking place in the clinical environment, making use of a vacant space such as a side room or empty ward area or the organization's own skills centre. The former have the advantage of creating a more realistic environment and an approach used by many mentors. In either setting the key to a successful learning experience is an enthusiastic, able and clinically credible facilitator.

TYPES OF SIMULATION

The type of simulation chosen for any particular learning experience will be dictated by the learning outcomes and facilities available and so must be carefully thought through beforehand. The following sections provide some examples of simulated scenarios you may like to be involved in or could use in your workplace or in a skills/simulation centre.

USE OF ROLE PLAY/ACTORS

A simulated clinical scenario can be created with people acting as the patient/client, and/or in some cases a relative. The 'actors' may be professional actors or a standardized patient (SP). SPs are usually volunteers who have been prepared for various roles. More usually the 'actors' will be colleagues; ideally they should not be someone with whom the student is very familiar. It is very difficult for the student to relate to someone as a patient when they are in fact known to them, such as the ward sister or a university lecturer and this detracts from the realism of the learning experience. Preparation of the actor whether they be professionals, SPs or colleagues is essential. They need to be clear about the student's learning outcomes and avoid any tendency to overact or ad lib. When using actors one of the key learning objectives is usually related to communication skills and the 'patient' can be primed to exhibit certain behaviours or ask particular questions but should react as realistically as possible to what the student actually does or says.

KEY POINT

If you use actors during a simulation exercise then prepare them beforehand on how to stay in character. You may like to consider giving them a detailed synopsis of who they are, perhaps even based on a 'real' patient they can identify with. This will be easier if they are not known to the student.

MIXED TASK TRAINER/ACTOR

Using this approach an actor can be used in conjunction with a training manikin or task trainer such as a catheterization model or venepuncture/cannulation arm. This allows the student to practise a potentially hazardous technique safely but in the context of a patient situation (see Case study 13.1)

Case study 13.1 *A student reflects on her experience of simulated learning*

'Last semester I was required to simulate the care I would give to a patient who was a diabetic and required an injection of insulin. When I went into the room it all seemed so real I actually forgot it was a simulation. There was an actor dressed in a hospital gown sitting in a chair. In my scenario they were a newly diagnosed diabetic and I needed to give a subcutaneous injection of insulin. There was even an injectable pad taped to the actor so I could really demonstrate my injection technique. My lecturer was standing off to the side watching and listening to everything I did. I had to demonstrate that I could give the medication correctly, communicate with the patient, answer questions and explain exactly what I was doing. At the end of the simulation I got feedback about how I did from my lecturer and we went through it step by step so I could see how to improve next time. I found it a brilliant learning experience.'

For example a student could be required to simulate catheterization technique by communicating with an actor but performing the actual task on a catheterization model. The learning activity would require the student to demonstrate the following:

- correct checking and preparation of all equipment
- gaining the patient's consent and providing adequate explanation
- answer the patient questions knowledgeably and in a way that will help to allay anxiety
- recognize if at any point further assistance is needed
- demonstrate safe and effective catheterization technique.

USE OF PATIENT SIMULATORS

There are many patient simulators on the market, some highly sophisticated and capable of producing highly realistic physiological responses that might be exhibited by a patient in a variety of states of health and illness. These are best suited to creating a scenario where the main objective is for the students to assess, observe, interpret and act on physiological changes that cannot be recreated in an actor. The addition of a 'patient voice' to the manikin enables the students to verbally interact with the patient. For example, a patient simulator can be set up as a postoperative patient (intravenous fluids running, catheter, wounds, drains and dressing in situ, oxygen in place). The patient simulator can be used to recreate signs of shock due to blood loss.

This kind of simulation can be resource intensive; someone is needed to operate the simulator and voice. This could be, but is not necessarily, the same person. In many cases it is helpful to have someone other than the person facilitating the simulation to be the person who is called upon to help. The more realistic you can make the simulation exercise the better the learning experience for the student. If you are undertaking a simulation exercise in practice consider having the actual person involved (e.g. the ward sister who would be called in a real-life situation) as this makes it all the more real. In addition to this you may chose to have other actors taking on other roles, for example as other patients or relatives who are either present or on the telephone.

The student must demonstrate:

- full systematic ABCDE assessment of the patient
- interpret and act upon the findings of the assessment appropriately
- document findings and seek appropriate help
- communicate with the patient and/or relative throughout in a manner that is knowledgeable and reassuring
- provide a clear, concise and relevant handover to the relevant member of staff.

All these examples of simulated experiences allow students to practise their skills and apply knowledge to patient care in a realistic and contextualized way. This approach can prepare them for similar situations in the real world of practice. This also allows assessment of and feedback on skills and knowledge in a way that is risk-free to patients and the student.

ARE YOU AND YOUR AREA PREPARED FOR SIMULATED LEARNING?

Before you start to use simulation within your mentoring role, whether in the clinical area or in an educational establishment you must ensure that you have prepared both yourself and the learning environment.

OPPORTUNITIES FOR SIMULATION

You should start by asking yourself why you would like to use simulation as an approach to learning. Some key questions include:

- What aspects of practice learning will we be using simulation for?

- Why is simulation useful here?
- What is the outcome or level of practice activity that we want the student to perform?

No doubt you will be able to identify a number quite quickly. For example, simulation is easily adaptable and a great learning experience for the following types of situations:

- patient assessment
- injection technique and other key skills
- communication skills
- basic life support.

Activity 13.1 asks you to explore this further.

Activity 13.1 Opportunities for simulated learning

Take some time to think about an aspect of practice where simulation could be used in your clinical area. Try to think how you would plan this session. You might like to separate this plan into categories:

- How many students will you have?
- Where is the simulation taking place? In trust/clinical area or in an educational establishment?
- What are your learning outcomes?
- What behaviours/actions are you expecting from students as part of the session?
- If some students are observing – what else will they be doing at that time?
- What resources do you have and which other staff are available to help?

PLANNING EFFECTIVE SIMULATION

The simulated learning environment needs to be as realistic as possible, so what is learnt and rehearsed is transferred easily into future practice. Within the clinical area it may be relatively easier to recreate a realistic environment as they will already be readily equipped with appropriate resources. Remember that empty wards and clinical areas are ideal venues for simulation as they can be quickly transformed into a realistic clinical environment.

Within a university simulation will require careful planning and sufficient resources to 'mock up' a convincing clinical setting. Planning will need to start early, so that equipment and supplies are available in good time.

On any manikin or human actor used within the simulation a range of recipes and procedures can be incorporated to mimic appropriate clinical situations or conditions such as bleeding, fake vomit, malaena, pus, etc. This practice is often referred to in literature and simulator user guides as ''moulage'. For access to tips and useful recipes for 'moulage' you can go to a number of websites, which include www.meti.com or www.laerdal.com.

> **KEY POINT**
>
> Closed wards can be ideal venues for simulation exercises; however, you must ensure that clear notices are put on all entry doors to ensure that real staff, patients and visitors within the organization do not wander in unexpectedly.

PREPARING TEACHING/CLINICAL COLLEAGUES

Before commencing the simulation session, you should discuss and agree both the learning outcomes and the session with any other colleagues who will be involved. During this discussion it is important that any constraints or concerns are acknowledged and that there is a realistic approach to what can be achieved in the session. Discuss and agree how time will be distributed throughout the session, ensuring that there is enough time for debriefing at the end, as this is where much of the learning takes place. Outline the learning resources/material (i.e. patient histories/scripts, etc. that will be required for the simulation) and agree who will be preparing this ahead of the session. Ensure all clinical/teaching staff involved are familiar with the plan, environment and equipment prior to the session. Having a trial run without students is very useful and supportive for those staff new to simulation, if there is time.

> **KEY POINT**
>
> When planning your first simulation exercise try to keep it simple and of short duration. This will minimize the amount of planning and organization required and allow you to build slowly upon success without becoming disheartened.

PREPARING THE STUDENTS

In order for the simulation session to have the maximum impact on student learning, it is important to ensure that students are prepared. Information can be made available regarding the scenario/patient and associated practice issues ahead of the session. This will ensure that students can prepare for the session by reviewing appropriate theory and practice guidelines and that they have some idea what will be expected of them during the simulation. If high-fidelity simulators are being used as part of the session, time must be allocated prior to the simulation to familiarize students with what the simulator can and cannot do, so that they know how to relate to it once it becomes 'their patient'.

USING A SIMULATION PLANNING TOOL

To ensure that all aspects of the planning are adequately addressed prior to the session it may be useful to have a planning tool template that all staff involved in simulation can refer to or use. An example of this is provided in Box 13.1.

PREPARATION OF STUDENTS PRIOR TO SESSION

Before you can commence a simulated learning activity you will need to check that students have completed the necessary tutorials or online programmes related to the topic area. For example, when creating a simulated subcutaneous injection exercise, as outlined in Box 13.2, you should ensure students have prior knowledge of:
- subcutaneous injection technique
- infection control
- hand washing
- drug administration
- health and safety in practice (e.g. disposal of sharps).

At the start of the session, ground rules will need to be agreed within the group – these may include aspects such as:
- positively supporting each other during the simulation
- not overtly criticizing each other during the simulation
- agreeing whether the facilitator can be asked for information during the simulation
- agreeing whether students can ask for 'time out/pause' if they want to stop the simulation.

Having ground rules such as these will encourage students to feel less anxious during the simulation, so that they can view it as a learning opportunity rather than an 'examination'. Students will also benefit from having a very clear scenario to work from as this will provide the necessary background from which they will enter the simulation event. An example scenario is provided in Box 13.3.

Box 13.1 Template/checklist for designing a simulation session

Date/Time of session:	**Title of session:**
Number of students:	

Learning outcomes for session:

Simulation scenario which would provide the desired physiology/Outline of storyboard

Identify resources needed/provided – time/staff, equipment, expertise?

Supporting material required/suggested	Provided?
Storyboard for students ahead of session – can be posted on virtual learning environment or in a teaching pack	Yes/No
Facilitator's notes, including a full version of the scenario and the behaviours/responses/actions you expect of the students	Yes/No
Information for the 'patient', whether that is the person providing the voice of the simulator, or the 'actor' who will be the patient	Yes/No
A full equipment list and, if using the simulators, information of the scenario needed	Yes/No
A checklist related to student behaviour/actions/responses expected	Yes/No
Activity identified for students waiting their turn for simulation	Yes/No
Time allocated format for debriefing/feedback	Yes/No
Students provided with a reflection/action plan sheet for inclusion in their portfolio	Yes/No
Evaluation tool developed/included	Yes/No

Box 13.2 Facilitating a simulation session for a subcutaneous injection

Learning outcomes

In this simulation session the student will be expected to:

- demonstrate safe practice in relation to administering a subcutaneous injection
- use communication skills to acknowledge the patient's feelings
- provide the patient with accurate information regarding the subcutaneous injection
- demonstrate professional behaviour throughout the procedure

Resources required

- sink area/alcohol hand rub
- receiver/insulin needle
- sterile water/labelled insulin
- male simulated patient/actor sat in hospital bed with skin tone injection pad (with metal backing) strapped to abdomen
- pyjamas
- name band
- drugs chart
- sharps bin
- curtains/screen
- gloves to be available

Box 13.3 Patient scenario

Michael is a 25-year-old single man who is a recently diagnosed diabetic. He has been admitted to hospital following a collapse during a football match. His diabetes is currently being stabilized with subcutaneous insulin. He is sitting in a bed on the medical ward. Insulin is to be administered as per prescription chart. You have five minutes to complete the procedure.

INFORMATION FOR SIMULATED PATIENT

If you are going to use actors in a simulation exercise then it is very important for them to understand their role and what is expected of them during the activity. For example, they may need to 'act' a certain way: angry, anxious, in pain, confused. Any actor involved in simulation will

---

Box 13.4 Scenario information for simulated patient

Past medical history

You have recently been diagnosed as a diabetic – you are struggling to control the diabetes with your diet

History of your present illness

You collapsed while playing football. You have not eaten since a curry late last night and you had a few beers

Behaviour

- You don't like doctors or hospital
- You feel 'awful' and don't want to be 'messed around'
- You are very impatient and just want to get home
- You wince loudly when the injection is given – and shout out 'is that your first time!'

Questions and prompts

- Answer student questions but show you are irritated by them
- Ask why you need the injection
- Be defensive when answering any questions about your life style and diet

---

need some clear instructions on the types of behaviour they might need to display and also some background about past health history and current health state. In Box 13.4 there is an example of the type of information that an actor for the scenario described earlier may require.

FEEDBACK FORMS

During the simulation sessions, you will need to complete a feedback sheet in relation to the range of student behaviours expected within this session. This form should include assessment of aspects of communication skills, professional behaviour, technical skills and health and safety considerations (see Case study 13.2). Examples of forms that can be used will be considered in the section on debriefing, later in this chapter.

In addition to feedback from the facilitator of the session, it is useful for the simulated patient to give formal feedback on how they felt the student did, especially commenting on their communication skills. This makes the role of simulated patient much more meaningful for the actor and it is an ideal way to get service user input into health care curriculum and student assessment.

Case study 13.2 *A student speaks of her experience of feedback following simulation*

'After the injection technique session I was pleased with the feedback I got, I didn't do everything perfectly but it showed that I was moving in the right direction. Rather than just going through the motions I had to use some initiative and communicate with the patient at the same time. The purpose of why I undertake this training and what I should be capable of doing as a result of it really hit me during this session as the simulated patient asked me so many questions while I was doing the injection. Now that I have moved on to yet another scenario it is becoming even clearer how important it is to take all variables into account and that with each passing week I'm gaining more knowledge and skills which complement each other. I will be able to use the feedback to improve my ability to be a competent nurse in the future.'

KEY POINT

It is useful for simulated patients within a simulation to deliver feedback while they are in character. Actors should be prepared for how to give this feedback, for example, how to respond to good practice and poor practice.

When organizing a simulated learning exercise you will want it to run smoothly with no major problems and difficulties. If you plan well for the event then there is a good chance that it will run according to plan. However, the reality is that sometimes it is the opposite of this that actually takes place. It's a good idea therefore to identify what potential problems might occur during a simulated learning exercise so systems can be put in place to prevent problems before they arise.

Case study 13.3 outlines an extreme example of a poor simulation exercise. In this scenario various factors contributed to the end result. The main failing was that the facilitator failed to prepare:

- themselves
- the technician
- the students.

As a direct result the session had no clear focus and no clear goals. Frequent interruptions and explanations made the learning experience

Case study 13.3 *A clinical educator's experience of simulation*

Mary is a clinical educator in a large teaching hospital. She decides to use a skills lab in the hospital to undertake a simulated learning session for pre-registration students currently on placement. Six students are asked to attend the skills lab but are given very little information about what to expect.

Mary is very busy and has very little time to prepare for the session. It takes her far longer than expected to prepare the scenario for the simulation and collect the clinical resources from the wards. Mary is not too sure what the high-fidelity patient simulator can do and decides to rely on the technician who will be running the simulator.

When the students arrive for the simulation session Mary notices that they are wearing their normal clothes and are not in uniform. They are very interested in the patient simulator and what it can do, but are also a bit nervous because they have not seen it before. In pairs they each take part in one of three simulations. The technician is not entirely clear what Mary wants to do throughout the simulation and has not been provided with the scenario. The simulation session is constantly interrupted by the students and the technician having to ask Mary questions and seek clarification about what the simulator can and can't do. Mary spends most of her time prompting the students to do things and at times has to halt the simulation altogether in order to give instructions. Not all of the equipment that the students need is available during the simulation. At the end of the session all six students comment to Mary that they have learnt very little and do not feel the simulation was realistic. Mary decides that simulation is no good for student learning and decides to never do it again.

unrealistic and frustrating for everyone involved. No one is expecting your simulation session/experience to be perfect; however, as a mentor you should be striving to create a positive learning experience and environment for all students. In order to do this through simulation you will need to put some time and effort into planning the simulation exercise to ensure that it runs smoothly and is as 'real' as possible.

KEY POINT

You might like to consider developing your own 'simulation' checklist that covers the essential elements of planning and facilitation within your organization.

PERSONAL PREPARATION

Assuming that you work in a clinical area that is suitable for simulation, the next step is to ensure that you are personally prepared for your role as a facilitator. Once again, you cannot assume that this will all just fall into place once you have observed a simulation session, and being personally prepared is your own responsibility – no-one can or should be expected to do this for you.

CONSIDER YOUR SKILLS IN RELATION TO FACILITATING LEARNING

In facilitation, the emphasis moves from teacher-centred to student-centred learning. This takes the pressure off you, as your role is in enabling and encouraging the learner to discover what they need to know and guiding them to the acquisition of that knowledge rather than knowing it all yourself. This can be quite challenging but what is more important is the mentor–student relationship, which allows the student to feel comfortable and able to make mistakes without ridicule.

If doing this with a group you need to consider group dynamics and create an atmosphere that promotes and allows safety, trust, enjoyment, listening, sharing and even non-participation, which are all important elements of effective facilitation. Whilst personal growth for all students is believed to be promoted by encouraging listening and sharing, ideally no value judgement is placed on non-contribution of students. Valuing and sharing the contributions of students in this way will encourage participation and therefore promote learning.

Preparation for your role as a facilitator and gaining further experience is important. You may have covered facilitation skills during your mentorship course or in a teaching course. Having completed this it is useful to take the opportunity to observe or assist with a simulation session to develop and refine your skills as part of your own professional development within a safe environment. Even experienced teachers with many hours of facilitation are expected to engage in peer review of their teaching practice. As facilitation can be considered as quite a demanding and intense process, leading to occasional discomfort, anxiety and insecurity, preparation and support for the role is crucial to the creation of a successful learning environment. If there is insufficient preparation for your role and a lack of opportunity to reflect on the effectiveness of your facilitation skills, this can result in an awkward teaching session that is little more than a string of orchestrated techniques.

Before and after simulation session

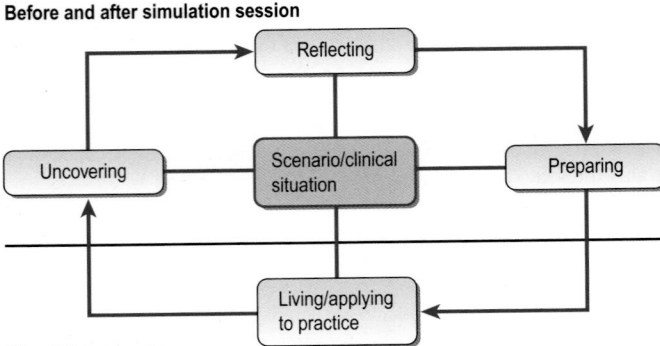

Simulation experience

Figure 13.1 Learning through simulation.

Some trusts/clinical areas encourage staff to participate in simulation activities either within the Trust or at the local university. This may even be included as part of a mentorship course. In other areas this is taken further with the opportunity to attend 'train the trainer' programmes related to the use of simulation.

The opportunity for you to develop your facilitation skills through supporting a simulation session will allow you to 'grow and develop' as a mentor and practitioner at the same time as supporting the 'growth and development' of students you come into contact with. While the actual simulation experience is a valuable learning opportunity (Figure 13.1), the real growth and development will come through your preparation for the simulation and then reflection on your strengths and weaknesses as a facilitator.

KEY POINT

Consider doing a 'mock' simulation exercise with your colleagues before inviting students to take part. This should iron out any practical issues such as availability of resources and the role of actors. It can also help to settle nerves so everyone involved is confident when it comes to the real thing.

If specific training on simulation is not available in your area, take the opportunity to find out what your students are doing at the university. Find out what simulation scenarios are part of their programme and help prepare and maintain student resources in your area to support this learning. If you get the chance, go and observe simulation taking place at work or in the local university and once you feel confident ask to take part.

DEBRIEFING AS PART OF SIMULATION

Discussion after the simulation is an important aspect of the learning process, and an essential element of the simulation exercise. For this reason debriefing after simulation should never be treated as dispensable or unnecessary. The purpose of debriefing after simulation is to:

- help the student to reflect on and analyse their actions
- assist the student to evaluate their own performance
- assist the student to evaluate their understanding of the clinical situation
- assist the student to evaluate how to improve their practice.

Before the simulation exercise you should have taken time to personally prepare yourself and the student for the simulation; identifying and reinforcing learning outcomes. The same consideration needs to be given to where, how and when you will debrief.

Generally debriefing occurs after the simulation. If you are unable to guarantee free uninterrupted time immediately after the simulation exercise you should identify a time to meet as soon as possible after. It is essential that you gain the trust of your student early in your relationship, as you will rely on this for the feedback to be valued. Debriefing is a facilitator-led approach to enable participants to review facts, thoughts, impressions and reactions to a prepared situation.

You might be required to use your skill in debriefing to empathize and reduce any stress your student may have encountered. The techniques employed need to take into account your student's individual learning styles. Remember that adults learn best when regular feedback and encouragement are provided, giving the all important progress check for the student. Debriefing is therefore an important aspect within the learning process, which helps the student to grow professionally.

Feedback after a simulation exercise will provide an opportunity to practise your active listening skills. Beware that your own views, feelings and opinions do not dominate the feedback event. You will need to indicate that you are interested and reinforce the value of the student's views and opinions. You may find it useful to follow a recognized model of reflection when debriefing after a simulation exercise. There are a number of different reflective models to choose from if you do wish to do this. The key is

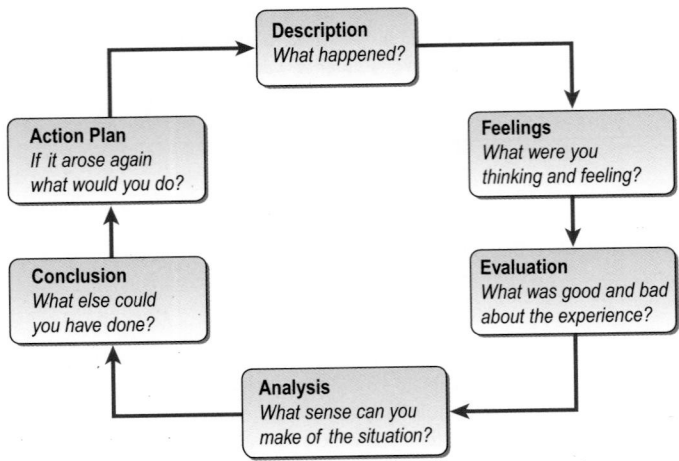

Figure 13.2 From Gibbs (1988) model of reflection with kind permission of OCSLD, Oxford Brookes University.

choosing a model that you are comfortable and familiar with, the most commonly used is the Gibbs (1988) model of reflection (Figure 13.2).

PLANNING FOR FEEDBACK

You should never undertake a simulation exercise until you have clearly thought about the learning outcomes and the competency the student is required to demonstrate. It is useful to design a simple tick sheet that outlines the various areas of competence that you want the student to develop with areas for comment and short notes (Box 13.5). You can then use these comments and notes as a basis for feedback after the session. Your feedback should take account of specific client care demonstrated in the simulation and stage of the programme your student is on.

It may also be possible to video record the simulation exercise. Alternatively, you may be able to get the student or group of students to use the tick/comment sheet on each other. This can be a powerful way to develop reflective skills and contribute to effective feedback; however, you will need to remember that some aspects of peer assessment can provoke anxiety if the peer group are close working colleagues or friends. Here, your knowledge of the students will help.

Box 13.5 Example feedback sheet

Simulation Feedback Sheet

Student name:

Date:

Expected behaviours	0	1	2	3	4	5	Comment
Personal professional presentation							
Applies alcohol gel/washes hands at appropriate times							
Communicates and assesses level of patient consciousness and pain							
Systematically assesses vital signs and fluid balance							
Observes wound sites							
Interprets vital signs correctly							
Documents/charts information accurately							
Communicates findings							
Demonstrates/discusses basic knowledge and understanding of the importance of post operative observations							

General comments:

Signed:

Name:

The decision of how you would like to design debriefing following simulation is clearly in your hands. You should always remember that there is a tension between making the student responsible for their own learning and ensuring maximum learning. Your understanding of the learning that needs to be met underpins all preparation. Certainly simulation undertaken within a course should show specifically identified intended learning outcomes; these are commonly included in the course module study guide. This should mean that the student is aware of what they should be learning and be making a plan as to how they will do this, under your guidance and expertise.

DELIVERING FEEDBACK

It is a good idea to start the feedback event by asking the student to reflect on how they feel they preformed during the simulation exercise. If you have more than one student ensure that the person who starts talking first is not seen to be the most valued. Often a stronger/more confident student can dominate the feedback and other participants can become disillusioned very quickly if this happens. Each student needs to be given the chance to discuss their view of their performance. Allow the student to state what they would alter and improve on if they were to do the exercise again. The key is to enhance critical thinking and problem solving, enabling the student to learn from their successes and identify what areas require improvement. This type of reflection will show you if the student has insight into their own abilities, and how they might progress and develop their skills.

POSITIVE FEEDBACK

Always begin a debriefing session with some positive feedback! At best the student will have a good idea if they have completed their task in the time you have scheduled. If this has taken place then you can congratulate them on their ability to undertake the exercise in 'real time' and reflect with them on how this meets what is expected from them at their stage of training. You can also congratulate them on their professional appearance and communication with the patient and each other. These aspects are important to record and value on the feedback sheet for future reference.

Thoughtful discussion allows the student to sort out events and interpret what happened and why. Sometimes a student will lack insight into their capabilities, and therefore your feedback should be reinforcing the student's confidence in themself. Students also find that individual/ small group feedback allows some enlightenment so don't be afraid of delivering feedback to groups as well as individuals. Try to be constructive towards the end of the feedback, you will need to help each student identify a progression plan, what the student needs to 'do' to progress and develop. While some students will have ideas on how to progress themselves, others will rely on you for guidance and advice.

STUDENTS' ATTITUDES TO SIMULATION

It is quite common for students to comment on how nervous they feel being observed, often telling you this before the simulation starts. You may even find that some students exacerbate their anxiety in order to gain sympathy! Your ability to make a student feel at ease before, during and after a simulation exercise is crucial. On occasions you might need to step in and interrupt the simulation to help the student relax before continuing on otherwise it may not achieve the learning planned (Case study 13.4).

Case study 13.4 A mentor speaks of her experience in a simulation exercise

'Last year I had the opportunity of going to the local university and taking part in a simulation exercise with a group of second-year adult branch students. The tutor had set the session up really well and I thought it was a really realistic way of getting the students to participate in a drug round. My role was to act as a mentor supervising a student doing a drug round. There were other actors playing the role of patients. One student in particular found the exercise very difficult. I felt that he had not prepared very well and was very unsure of how to perform the drug calculations. At one stage he stopped and said' 'I could do this if you were not watching me'. I had been told to stay in character so gave him the same response that I would if we really were on a ward in the middle of a round. I explained that the NMC requires a mentor to supervise students administering medications. At this point I got a different excuse; his response was that 'I can normally do this, but I can't understand why not today'. When we finished the drug round I was able to do a formal reflection with this student and it became clear that he was genuinely disappointed with his performance, and had been using excuses to try to mask the fact that his knowledge on drug calculations was poor. We were able to reflect that a function of the simulation was to highlight any areas where improvements were needed, and from my point of view the exercise had been a success rather than a failure. Once he realized that it was his learning and not my opinion that mattered we made real progress.'

It's not always possible, but you should try to prevent the students from attempting to blame any poor performance during a simulation exercise on an independent issue. If you have checked that every student feels able to attempt the exercise, both in terms of their understanding of what they are required to achieve, and that they feel well enough/relaxed enough to go ahead; then these issues should not be used as the basis of an excuse following the exercise. Prior to the session commencing you should ask some simple and direct questions that will allow each student to declare confidentially the need for any reasonable adjustments they may require.

GETTING IT RIGHT

While there is no guarantee that planning and preparation will prevent all problems, it will assist in troubleshooting the most common areas where simulation does not go as well as expected. Get this right and there is every chance that the simulation exercise will be an invaluable learning tool (Case study 13.5). Successful simulation can result in advanced preparation for practice learning opportunities as well as providing a student with alternative learning experiences while on practice placement.

Case study 13.5 A student reflects on simulation

'Thinking about the simulation, I realized that it wasn't about trying to remember what came next like a list in my head, but rather how the result of one investigation would prompt your next move and that practical implications guide you through the motions instead. The purpose of why we undertake all this study and what we should be capable of doing really hit me that day. Now we have to move onto yet another scenario it is becoming clearer how important it is to take all variables into account and that with each passing week we are gaining more knowledge and skills which complement each other. The links between theory and practice are becoming clearer and I am often encouraged to learn more in my own time about the physiology related to the simulation. The confidence I am gaining as a nurse is growing as a result of the simulation sessions.'

TOP TIPS

- Ensure everyone involved in the simulation has been prepared for their role and has had staff development related to facilitating simulation.
- Ensure that learning outcomes/expected student behaviours/time of simulation session are outlined ahead of the session.
- Agree and prepare the scenario/storyboard for simulation ahead of the session.
- Provide information sheets/packs for 'patients or actors' that are participating in the simulation.
- Ensure you have full equipment lists and are provided with 'set up' instructions.
- Allow adequate time following the session for debriefing and feedback.

References

Gibbs G (1988) *Learning by Doing: A Guide to Teaching and Learning Methods.* Further Education Unit, Oxford Polytechnic, Oxford.

Maran, NJ and Glavin RJ (2003) Low- to high-fidelity simulation – a continuum of medical education. *Medical Education* 37 (Suppl. 1):22–28.

CHAPTER 14

EVALUATING THE LEARNING EXPERIENCE

Chapter Aims

The purpose of this chapter is to explore strategies for evaluating the quality of the learning experience for students and your success as a mentor. After reading this chapter you will be able to:

- Explain why evaluation is important.
- Identify strategies for evaluating the student experience in practice.
- Identify your own strengths and weaknesses as a mentor.

WHY EVALUATION IS IMPORTANT

Just as it is important to evaluate the care you deliver to patients and clients it is also important to evaluate the quality of a student's learning experience with you, not only to determine whether they had an effective learning experience themselves but also whether you were effective in your role as a mentor. You might question whether you can have one without the other, but feedback from students suggests that they can achieve their learning objectives despite having a mentor who has been unsupportive or ineffective. However, where students have a good mentor (and we'll discuss what makes a good mentor later) there is no question that their learning will be enhanced. Evaluation therefore will enable you to improve your mentorship skills and so the learning experience for future students.

> **KEY POINT**
>
> Evaluation is key for improvement. Without evaluation you risk making the same mistakes over and over again.

WHEN TO EVALUATE

Evaluation is often seen as something that takes place at the end of a programme or in this case a placement. However, evaluation should be ongoing, you certainly wouldn't wait until the end of a patient's stay to evaluate whether your care had been effective, nor should you with a student!

Just as you give feedback at regular intervals to your student it is also helpful to get feedback from them on the support you and other staff are providing them and whether their objectives and learning needs are being met. This gives the student an opportunity to raise any concerns which can be managed rather than waiting until the end when it is too late. Sometimes you may not be able to change what the student is unhappy about but the fact that you have asked and listened will go a long way with the student and it will have identified something that the placement can work on for the future.

WHAT TO EVALUATE

Before deciding how you wish to evaluate the student experience you need to decide exactly what it is you wish to evaluate. Are you looking at the overall experience or do you want to focus on something specific? For example, you may have introduced something new such as an orientation booklet for students and want to focus on that or you may have introduced new learning activities for students and want to know if they were valued by the students. Potential areas for evaluation are:

- the student's experience of the placement
- the quality of the placement as a learning environment
- your own experience of mentoring the student
- your role as a mentor.

Each of these areas will overlap to a certain extent. A student's experience of their placement will be heavily influenced by the quality of the mentorship they receive. Equally, a placement that is a poor environment for learning will impact on your ability to mentor effectively and the quality of a student's learning experience.

KEY POINT

The main areas that you evaluate should always be focused on the standards of mentorship.

THE STUDENT'S EXPERIENCE OF THE PLACEMENT

Students are required by the university to evaluate their experience in practice and this contributes to the university quality assurance processes. Student evaluation is undertaken by the university and should be fed back to the placement providers at regular intervals. There is no standard evaluation tool, so each university will have a different approach to this and the type of questions they ask. If you have never seen the evaluations of your area by students you should first check with your manager whether they have received them and failing that contact the link lecturer attached to your area who should be able to provide you with a copy or show you how to access them if available on-line. The areas that the questions are likely to cover are:

- preparation and orientation to the placement
- mentor support
- learning opportunities and experience
- assessment process
- learning climate (what the area is like overall for learning).

An example of the type of questions that may be asked by a university regarding a student's experience of their placement can be found in Table 14.1.

THE QUALITY OF THE PLACEMENT AS A LEARNING ENVIRONMENT

EDUCATIONAL AUDITS

Universities are required by the NMC to undertake an educational audit of all areas that they use for student placements. The rationale for this is to ensure that the placement has sufficient resources to support the number of students who will be placed there at any one time and that it can provide the appropriate learning opportunities to enable the students to meet specified learning outcomes (i.e. your placement may be appropriate for students at any point on a programme or only appropriate for a specific part of a programme). However, an audit also enables the university and practice to identify specific areas in a placement that the staff there may need help and support to maintain, improve or develop to ensure the quality of the learning environment for students as well as for identifying areas of good practice that can be disseminated to other placement areas.

The audits are usually undertaken in partnership with the staff in the placement and will take place every one or two years. Both the university and the placement will retain a copy of the completed audit so you should be able to get a copy of your most recent audit very easily. As with student evaluations of practice each university will have a different format

Table 14.1 Sample student evaluation form for practice placements

	Strongly agree	Agree	Disagree	Strongly disagree
Preparation and orientation I was orientated to the placement including, fire regulations, health & safety issues, resuscitation equipment policy & routines on my first day				
Preparation and orientation The practice area was expecting me				
Mentor and teacher support I was allocated a mentor at the start of my placement				
Mentor and teacher support My mentor welcomed me, was friendly and approachable and treated me as an individual				
Mentor and teacher support My mentor was keen to support and facilitate my learning				
Mentor and teacher support My mentor was knowledgeable about my course and the assessment scheme				
Mentor and teacher support I worked with my mentor a minimum of 40% of the time				
Mentor and teacher support Planned absence of my mentor was covered with a co-mentor				
Mentor and teacher support My mentor provided a menu of learning opportunities and helped me to organize the learning experiences				
Mentor and teacher support I was made aware of the contact person from my university and how to contact them				

Statement					
Learning in practice assessment I was guided in clarifying the learning objective for the placement					
Learning in practice assessment I had opportunities to observe skilled practitioners delivering care					
Learning in practice assessment I had opportunities to participate in delivery of care under guidance and supervision					
Learning in practice assessment I received regular feedback on my performance					
Learning in practice assessment The learning opportunities were structured and coordinated to help me develop competencies					
Learning in practice assessment I had opportunities to discuss and reflect on issues relating to practice and theory					
Learning in practice assessment I had opportunities to attend teaching sessions where available, undertake visits and meet other practitioners relevant to the placement area					
Learning in practice assessment Practice assessment criteria were explained to me					
Learning in practice assessment The assessment process and completion of documentation was appropriate and timely					
Learning climate Learning opportunities available were relevant to my learning outcomes					
Learning climate The staff attached great importance to the learning needs of students					

Continued

Table 14.1 Sample student evaluation form for practice placements—cont'd

	Strongly agree	Agree	Disagree	Strongly disagree
Learning climate All staff including students feel part of the health care team				
Learning climate There was a range of learning resources available in this placement				
Learning climate I was able and encouraged to ask questions				
Learning climate The provision of care reflects respect for privacy, dignity, cultural beliefs and evidence-based practice				
Learning climate The patient care needs really are given first priority				
Learning climate This was a good unit for my learning				

Based on the Student Evaluation form at Thames Valley University.

for their audit but it will include questions or statements against which the placement will be judged and are likely to cover:

- details of placement (name, address, telephone number, contact person)
- health and safety policies and procedures
- information about the learning environment, resources available and the learning opportunities available
- assessment of the area's capacity to take students, including whether related to modules the student is studying or year of their programme
- evidence of a live register of mentors
- evidence of approaches to teaching learning and assessment and supporting students in practice.

At the end of an educational audit document there is usually space for an action plan to remedy any areas that require improvement. By reviewing the audit you can identify where your placement area is meeting the expected standards and those areas that need improvement.

KEY POINT

Ask to look at the education audit for your practice area. It will typically be held by the manager and will highlight any particular areas for improvement to do with mentor and student support.

Other reports which might inform you about the quality of your area as a learning environment are:

- internal audits, e.g. numbers of pressure sores, medication errors, staffing levels, infection rates
- Care Quality Commission reports (available at www.cqc.org.uk).

EVALUATING YOUR OWN EXPERIENCE

There are a number of different strategies that you can use to evaluate your own experience of mentoring and your effectiveness as a mentor. This section will look at four that you can use to either self-evaluate your own experience or gain feedback from others about your performance as a mentor.

SWOT ANALYSIS

SWOT stands for **S**trengths, **W**eaknesses, **O**pportunities and **T**hreats. It is a tool that can be used to examine both your own performance as a mentor and the area in which you work as a learning environment for students. Activity 14.1 requires you to undertake a SWOT analysis.

Activity 14.1 SWOT analysis

Think about students you have mentored over the last year and write a few notes under each of the headings listed below:

Strengths

What were the strong points of your mentorship? What did you do well?

Weaknesses

What were your weaknesses as a mentor? What could you have done better?

Opportunities

What opportunities are there to enable you to improve as a mentor?

Threats

What are the threats to you as a mentor? What stopped you mentoring as well as you would have wished with recent students?

REFLECTION

All students are required to reflect on their practice so asking you to reflect on your own practice as a mentor makes a lot of sense. It allows you to become familiar with the reflective models that they use and also to appreciate how challenging this can be at times but also how valuable. There are a range of reflective models or frameworks that you can use and it is worth trying several to see which one suits you best. If you are unfamiliar with them then it is probably a good idea to talk to the students you have or the link lecturer from their university to find out what models they use. Models can be circular in format or a list of questions that you answer but all have common elements:

- looking back on what happened
- examining thoughts and feelings about what happened
- identifying what went well and not so well
- identifying what you have learnt from the experience
- considering how you will respond to a similar situation in the future.

When reflecting you can choose a specific element of the mentoring relationship (e.g. giving feedback), a particular moment that went well or not so well (e.g. demonstrating a skill) or look at the whole period of mentorship with one student. It is useful to record your reflections in a journal. This allows you to look back over time to see what you have learnt and how you have developed. It is also a good way of picking up common themes. For example, you may find that you have similar problems with each student such as giving feedback, and this can focus your attention on an area in which you need to develop. Activity 14.2 takes you through a series of questions to help you reflect on a mentoring experience.

Activity 14.2 A checklist for personal reflection

Think back to a student you have recently mentored and answer the following questions about your experience of mentoring that student:

- How did you feel about the mentoring relationship between yourself and your student? What was good about it? What did you feel uncomfortable about?
- What went well during the mentoring episode? Why do think this was?
- What did not go well? Why do you think this was?
- What could you have done to have improved the situation?
- What have you learnt about yourself as a mentor from this mentoring episode?
- How will you use this new knowledge to improve your skills as a mentor for the future?

Look at the list above and congratulate yourself on your strengths. Consider the weaknesses. What can you do to strengthen these? Consider the opportunities – are you making the most of these? Look at the threats. What can you do personally to reduce them? You could develop this into a personal action plan to work on as part of your own professional development. You could also take it to your next Triennial Review meeting with your manager. If there are particular issues that you feel need action now that are impacting on the quality of student learning then discuss with your manager as soon as possible.

GUIDED REFLECTION

Reflective practice can be a solitary exercise and requires you to have a high degree of self-awareness and the ability to be critically honest about your actions and feelings. Sharing your reflections with another person can be helpful as another person can challenge your actions, feelings and assumptions and so help you to become more aware of your thoughts and behaviours.

> **KEY POINT**
>
> If possible, try to discuss the events of each practice placement with all staff regularly at team meetings. Issues can be highlighted and problems resolved very quickly if they are talked about openly and constructively.

STUDENT QUESTIONNAIRE

You might like to consider a brief questionnaire that you give students at the end of their placement with you. The challenge with this approach is that because the student knows that you will be reading the answers that they may not be as honest as they might when they answer a questionnaire which is anonymous or completed once they are back at the university. To gain the most honest answers it is best to ask the student to complete the questionnaire after you have completed their practice assessment document and ask them to return it to you in a sealed envelope. The shorter the questionnaire the more likely that a student is to complete it, so consider what you think are the important areas you want feedback on. You can use the feedback you receive to carry out a self-evaluation of the placement as a whole to identify the areas that you achieved, and also the areas that improvements need to be made. Box 14.1 provides an example of some of the information you might like to receive feedback on.

ANALYSING EVALUATIONS

Analysing student evaluations can be daunting and how you go about this will depend on how they are presented. Evaluations can be quantitative or qualitative or a mix of both. Examples of quantitative evaluations are a set of questions with:

- Yes or No answers – the total number of Yes answers and No answers are then calculated for each question.

Box 14.1 Feedback questionnaire from students

My mentor had planned for my arrival before the start of placement
Comments . . . .
. . . .

I was welcomed on my first day and orientated to the placement area
Comments . . . .
. . . .

My mentor conducted the initial interview in the first week
Comments . . . .
. . . .

My mentor reviewed all learning objectives during the first week and
assisted me to plan learning experiences
Comments . . . .
. . . .

My mentor provided me with regular verbal and written feedback
regarding my progress
Comments . . . .
. . . .

My mentor provided action/development plans where required
Comments . . . .
. . . .

My mentor reviewed all learning objectives with me at the midpoint of
the placement, providing verbal and written feedback as required
Comments . . . .
. . . .

My mentor conducted a final interview that provided me with feedback
related to all learning objectives I undertook during the placement
Comments . . . .
. . . .

My mentor completed a fair and accurate final assessment based on
evidence of continuous assessment
Comments . . . .
. . . .

My mentor provided me with an opportunity to give me feedback on
my mentor's performance
Comments . . . .
. . . .

My mentor provided a debrief opportunity for the placement
Comments . . . .
. . . .

● Likert scale – the student can answer the questions against a scale: e.g. strongly agree, agree, disagree, strongly disagree. The total number of answers for each of the points on the Likert scale can then be calculated for each question.

For each of the above you can add up the scores for each question from a set of student evaluations and see which questions score well and those that score less well. Those that score less well may be areas that your placement or you need to improve upon.

Qualitative evaluations give a student an opportunity to write comments in response to one or more questions. These answers can be more difficult to analyse as the quality of the answers will depend on the quality of the questions, the student's understanding of the question and their ability to give an answer that is succinct and clear.

The more evaluations you can collect the more valuable they are. One single evaluation tells you what that particular student felt, whereas a number of valuations allow you to see if there are any particular trends. Now try Activity 14.3.

Activity 14.3

Extract from a student evaluation

'I arrived on my first day but no-one was expecting me, although they quickly allocated me a mentor'

Consider why this may have occurred and jot down below:

What actions would you take for each of your answers above to ensure it didn't happen again?

Comments on Activity 14.3

Possible reasons you may have given are:

● the planned mentor being off sick/on annual leave/a different shift.
● an oversight by the manager of the placement.
● an error by the university in informing the placement that a student was coming.

If only one student evaluation states this as an issue then this may have been a one-off occurrence; however, if more than one student highlights this as an issue then there is clearly a problem regarding either the way mentors are allocated to students or the way that the university is informing the placement area when students will be coming to them.

Possible strategies to ensure this won't happen again are:

- allocating all students two mentors
- ensuring that at least one mentor is on duty on a student's first day
- ensuring mentors who are allocated a student are not due to take leave at the start of a student's placement with them
- identifying a specific person to be responsible for mentor allocations
- discussing with the university how allocations are communicated.

Whilst the majority of students praise their mentors and their placement experience there will be some students who will be less than happy with their experience. If you receive less than positive evaluations it is important to consider why this may be.

KEY POINT

If a student does evaluate your practice area as poor then try to account for why this might be. Don't be defensive, look for specific objective evidence to support the student evaluation.

LESSONS LEARNT

No-one likes to hear bad news and it is important not to take evaluations that are critical of you or the placement where you work too personally. Rather, consider what may have caused the student to be critical and whether they have justification for their comments. Reflect on whether there were any difficulties with particular students or in the placement itself at the time that they were with you that may have led them to evaluate their experience negatively. Examples of factors that may lead to negative evaluations are:

- staff shortages impacting on the level of support and supervision offered to a student
- changes in service delivery (e.g. ward closing for Christmas, or changing its specialty)
- lack of understanding by mentors about the student's programme/ learning outcomes/needs/practice assessment document
- student was failed by their mentor.

The first two points should have been anticipated by the manager and actions taken in advance of students coming to the placement. Any changes to a placement or reductions in staffing levels should be communicated to the university in order that they can reconsider whether students should be allocated to you or whether students at a different stage of their programme are more suited. The third point is a failing by the mentors to fulfil their responsibility to ensure that they are up-to-date with the students' programme and practice assessment process by attending annual updates. The last point cannot be so easily anticipated but it is important to consider when a student has been failed and evaluates a placement negatively, whether they were supported appropriately during their placement and the assessment process was fair and just.

The feedback you receive from students will provide invaluable insight into your own mentoring performance. It can be a great way to find out how your mentoring is perceived by students. You may like to use your self-reflective checklist and the feedback from students to answer the following questions.

1. What aspects of mentoring do you excel in?
2. How can you share these aspects with others and encourage them to do likewise?
3. What aspects of mentoring do you not achieve or receive poor feedback on?
4. What can you do to strengthen you weaker areas?
5. Based on your last mentoring experience, what will you definitely do again?
6. Based on your last mentoring experience, what will you do differently?

KEY POINT

Share good mentoring practice with others in your team. If you are doing something particularly well then share this experience so others may learn from your expertise.

IMPROVING THE LEARNING ENVIRONMENT

Discussions with students about their practice experience when they return to the university reveals common threads on what has made a positive learning experience for them. The most important is the mentor. Students describe the good mentor as welcoming, supportive, willing, friendly and approachable. Elements that students report back that have made a good placement for them are:

- the student was expected and welcomed
- the mentor was interested in the student and the student felt part of the team
- the mentor was able to work regularly with the student
- the student was able to practise a range of skills
- information was available on how to prepare for the placement
- mentor (and staff) were seen as knowledgeable.

There are a number of activities that you could consider undertaking to make your area a positive learning environment for students most of which, once done, only need a small amount of time to keep them maintained. Examples of such activities include:

- sending out pre-placement letters to students to welcome them to the area
- ensuring your orientation pack is up-to-date and includes only useful information
- providing a student noticeboard with contact details and learning opportunities
- an easily accessible resource folder for mentors and students.

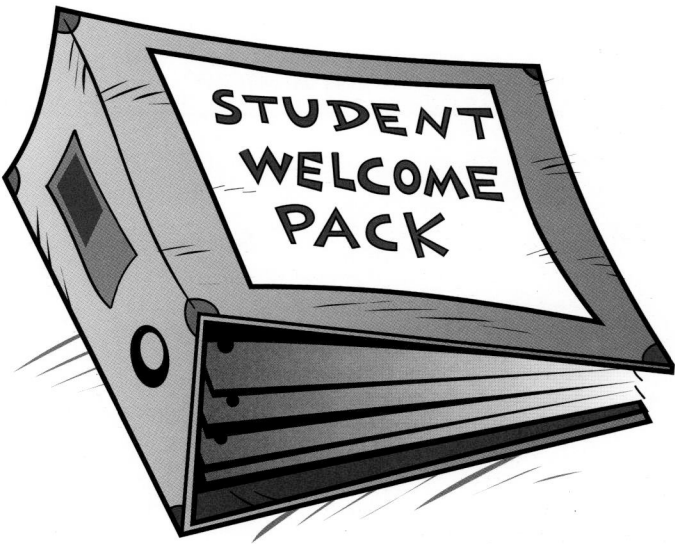

POSITIVE MENTORING

The best outcome from a practice placement is that both you and your student have had a positive, rewarding experience. Not only will you have had an opportunity for facilitating learning experiences, you will have made a valuable contribution as a gatekeeper to the profession. If experiences during the practice placement are less than satisfactory then it is important that you view these as an opportunity to improve, rather then lose motivation. Seek feedback about your mentoring skill from a wide variety of students and use this information to improve your own professionalism. Never stop striving towards being the best mentor you can possibly be.

TOP TIPS

- Ask to see the student evaluations about your placement twice a year so you can identify what is working well and what needs improving.
- Keep a reflective journal that records both the positive experiences and challenges you have with students; you can then use this at your triennial review.
- Share good practice with others. If an aspect of your mentoring has been positively evaluated then share this with your colleagues.

THE DEVELOPMENTAL FRAMEWORK TO SUPPORT LEARNING AND ASSESSMENT IN PRACTICE

From the NMC (2008) with permission of the Nursing and Midwifery Council

Domain: Establishing effective working relationships

Demonstrate effective relationship building skills sufficient to support learning, as part of a wider interprofessional team, for a range of students in both practice and academic learning environments

Stage 1 Nurses and midwives	Stage 2 Mentor	Stage 3 Practice teacher	Stage 4 Teacher
Work as a member of a multi-professional team, contributing effectively to team working	Demonstrate an understanding of factors that influence how students integrate into practice settings	Have effective professional and interprofessional working relationships to support learning for entry to the register and education at a level beyond initial registration	Demonstrate effective relationships with other members of the teaching teams in practice and academic settings based on mutual trust and respect
Support those who are new to the team in integrating into the practice learning environment	Providing ongoing and constructive support to facilitate transition from one learning environment to another	Be able to support students moving into specific areas of practice or a level of practice beyond initial registration, identifying their individual needs in moving to a different level of practice	Maintain appropriate supportive relationships with a range of students, mentors, practice teachers and other professionals
Act as a role model for safe and effective practice	Have effective professional and interprofessional working relationships to support learning for entry to the register	Support mentors and other professionals in their roles to support learning across practice and academic learning environments	Foster peer support and peer learning in practice and academic settings for all students
Develop effective working relationships based on mutual trust and respect			Support students to integrate into new environments and working teams to enhance access to learning

Domain: Facilitation of learning

Facilitate learning for a range of students, within a particular area of practice where appropriate, encouraging self-management of learning opportunities and providing support to maximize individual potential

Stage 1 Nurses and midwives	Stage 2 Mentor	Stage 3 Practice teacher	Stage 4 Teacher
Co-operate with those who have defined support roles contributing towards the Provision of effective learning experiences	Use knowledge of the student's stage of learning to select appropriate learning opportunities to meet individual needs	Enable students to relate theory to practice whilst developing critically reflective skills	Promote development of enquiring, reflective, critical and innovative approaches to learning
Share their own knowledge and skills to enable others to learn in practice settings	Facilitate the selection of appropriate learning strategies to integrate learning from practice and academic experience	Foster professional growth and personal development by use of effective communication and facilitation skills	Implement a range of learning and teaching strategies across a wide range of settings
	Support students in critically reflecting upon their learning experiences in order to enhance future learning	Facilitate and develop the ethos of interprofessional learning and working	Provide support and advice, with ongoing and constructive feedback to students, to maximize individual potential
			Co-ordinate learning within an interprofessional learning and working environment
			Facilitate integration of learning from practice and academic settings
			Act as a practice expert to support development of knowledge and skills for practice

Continued

Domain: Assessment and accountability

Assess learning in order to make judgements related to the NMC standards of proficiency for entry to the register or for recording a qualification at a level above initial registration

Stage 1 Nurses and midwives	Stage 2 Mentor	Stage 3 Practice teacher	Stage 4 Teacher
Work to the NMC Code for nurses and midwives in maintaining own knowledge and proficiency for safe and effective practice	Foster professional growth, personal development and accountability through support of students in practice	Set effective professional boundaries whilst creating a dynamic, constructive teacher–student relationship	Set and maintain professional boundaries that are sufficiently flexible for interprofessional learning
Provide feedback to others in learning situations and to those who are supporting them so that learning is effectively assessed	Demonstrate a breadth of understanding of assessment strategies and ability to contribute to the total assessment process as part of the teaching team	In partnership with other members of the teaching team use knowledge and experience to design and implement assessment frameworks	Develop, with others, effective assessment strategies to ensure that standards of proficiency for registration or recordable qualifications at a level beyond initial registration are met
	Provide constructive feedback to students and assist them in identifying future learning needs and actions. Manage failing students so that they may enhance their performance and capabilities for safe and effective practice or be able to understand their failure and the implications of this for their future	Be able to assess practice for registration and also at a level beyond that of initial registration	Support others involved in the assessment process, students, mentors and peers
	Be accountable for confirming that students have met or not met the NMC competencies in	Provide constructive feedback to students and assist them in identifying future learning needs and actions, manage failing students so that they may enhance their performance and capabilities for safe and effective practice or be able to understand their failure and the implications of this for their future	Provide constructive feedback to students and assist them in identifying future learning needs and actions, manage failing students so that they may enhance their performance and capabilities for safe and effective practice or be able to understand their failure and the implications of this for their future

| | | Be accountable for confirming that students have met or not met the NMC standards of proficiency in practice for registration at a level beyond initial registration and are capable of safe and effective practice | Be accountable for decisions related to fitness for practice for registration or recordable qualifications, underpinning such decisions with an evidence base derived from appropriate and effective monitoring of performance |
| | | | |

| | practice and as a signoff mentor confirm that students have met or not met the NMC standards of proficiency and are capable of safe and effective practice | | |

Domain: Evaluation of learning

Determine strategies for evaluating learning in practice and academic settings to ensure that the NMC standards of proficiency for registration or recording a qualification at a level above initial registration have been met

Stage 1 Nurses and midwives	Stage 2 Mentor	Stage 3 Practice teacher	Stage 4 Teacher
Contribute information related to those learning in practice, and about the nature of learning experiences, to enable those supporting students to make judgements on the quality of the learning environment	Contribute to evaluation of student learning and assessment experiences, proposing aspects for change resulting from such evaluation Participate in self- and peer evaluation to facilitate personal development and contribute to the development of others	Design evaluation strategies to determine the effectiveness of practice and academic experience accessed by students at both registration level and those in education at a level beyond initial registration Collaborate with other members of the teaching team to judge and develop learning, assessment, and support appropriate to practice and levels of education	Determine and use criteria for evaluating the effectiveness of learning environments, acting on findings, with others, to enhance quality Foster and participate in self- and peer evaluation to enable students to manage their own learning in practice and academic settings and to enhance personal professional development Evaluate the effectiveness of assessment strategies in

Continued

Domain: Evaluation of learning—Cont'd

Collect evidence on the quality of education in practice, and determine how well NMC requirements for standards of proficiency are being achieved

providing evidence to make judgements on fitness for practice

Report on the quality of practice and academic learning environments to demonstrate that NMC requirements have been met, particularly in relation to support of students and achievement of standards of proficiency

Domain: Create an environment for learning

Create an environment for learning, where practice is valued and developed, that provides appropriate professional and interprofessional learning opportunities and support for learning to maximize achievement for individuals

Stage 1 Nurses and midwives	Stage 2 Mentor	Stage 3 Practice teacher	Stage 4 Teacher
Demonstrate a commitment to continuing professional development to enhance own knowledge and proficiency Provide peer support to others to facilitate their learning	Support students to identify both learning needs and experiences that are appropriate to their level of learning Use a range of learning experiences, involving patients, clients, carers and the professional team, to meet defined learning needs	Enable students to access opportunities to learn and work within interprofessional teams Initiate the creation of optimum learning environments for students at registration level and for those in education at a level beyond initial registration	In partnership with others, opportunities for students to identify and access learning experiences that meet their individual needs Ensure such opportunities maintain the integrity of the student's professional role whilst respondin

Stage 1	Stage 2	Stage 3	Stage 4
Identify aspects of the learning environment which could be enhanced negotiating with others to make appropriate changes Act as a resource to facilitate personal and professional development of others	Work closely with others involved in education, in practice and academic settings, to adapt to change and inform curriculum development		practi… Determine with others, audit criteria against which learning environments may be judged for their effectiveness in meeting NMC requirements Support and develop others involved to ensure that learning needs are effectively met in a safe environment Explore and implement strategies for continuous quality improvement of the learning environment

Domain: Context of practice

Support learning within a context of practice that reflects health care and educational policies, managing change to ensure that particular professional needs are met within a learning environment that also supports practice development

Stage 1 Nurses and midwives	Stage 2 Mentor	Stage 3 Practice teacher	Stage 4 Teacher
Whilst enhancing their own practice and proficiency, a registered nurse or midwife, act as a role model to others to enable them to learn their unique professional role	Contribute to the development of an environment in which effective practice is fostered, implemented, evaluated and disseminated Set and maintain professional boundaries that are sufficiently	Recognize the unique needs of practice and contribute to development of an environment that supports achievement of NMC standards of proficiency	Support students in identifying ways in which policy impacts on practice Contribute effectively to processes of change and innovation, implementing new ways of working that maintain

Continued

Domain: Context of practice—Cont'd		
flexible for providing interprofessional care	Set and maintain professional boundaries, whilst at the same time recognizing the contribution of the wider interprofessional team and the context of care delivery	the integrity of professional roles
Initiate and respond to practice developments to ensure safe and effective care is achieved and an effective learning environment is maintained		Negotiate ways of providing support to students so that they can achieve their learning needs within the context of professional and interprofessional practice
	Support students in exploring new ways of working and the impact this may have on established professional roles	Act as a role model to enable students to learn professional responsibilities and how to be accountable for their own practice
		Adapt to change, demonstrating to students how flexibility may be incorporated whilst maintaining safe and effective practice

Domain: Evidence-based practice			
Apply evidence-based practice to their own work and contribute to the further development of such a knowledge and practice			
Stage 1 Nurses and midwives	Stage 2 Mentor	Stage 3 Practice teacher	Stage 4 Teacher
Further develop their evidence base for practice to support their own personal and	Identify and apply research and evidence-based practice to their area of practice	Identify areas of research and practice development based o[...]	Adva[...]

		interpretation of existing evidence	where appropr. and practice deve.
professional development and to contribute to the development of others	Contribute to strategies to increase or review the evidence base used to support practice	Use local and national health frameworks to review and identify developmental needs	Consider how evide. practice, involving patie. clients, carers and other members of the health and social care team, enhances care delivery and learning opportunities
	Support students in applying an evidence base to their own practice	Advance their own knowledge and practice in order to develop new practitioners, at both registration levels and education at a level beyond initial registration, to be able to meet changes in practice roles and care delivery	Empower individuals, groups and organizations to develop the evidence base for practice
		Disseminate findings from research and practice development to enhance practice and the quality of learning experiences	Disseminate findings from the research and practice development to enhance the quality of learning and care delivery and academic environments

Domain: Leadership

Demonstrate leadership skills for education within practice and academic settings

Stage 1 Nurses and midwives	Stage 2 Mentor	Stage 3 Practice teacher	Stage 4 Teacher
Use communication skills effectively to ensure that those in learning experiences understand their contribution and limitations to care delivery	Plan a series of learning experiences that will meet students' defined learning needs	Provide practice leadership and expertise in application of knowledge and skills based on evidence	Demonstrate effective communication skills to facilitate delivery of educational programmes leading to

Continued

Domain: Leadership—Cont'd

Be an advocate for students to support them accessing learning opportunities that meet their individual needs, involving a range of other professionals, patients, clients and carers	Demonstrate the ability to lead education on practice, working across practice and academic settings	registration or a recordable qualification
Prioritize work to accommodate support of students within their practice roles	Manage competing demands of practice and education related to supporting different practice levels of students	Initiate and lead programme development and review processes to enhance quality and effectiveness
Provide feedback about the effectiveness of learning and assessment in practice	Lead and contribute to the evaluation of effectiveness of learning and assessment in practice	Develop effective relationships with practice and academic staff involved in programme delivery to ensure clarity of contribution and strategies to respond to evaluation of learning experiences
		Demonstrate strategic vision for practice and academic development relevant to meeting NMC requirements
		Manage competing demands to ensure effectiveness of learning experiences for students
		Lead, contribute to, analyse and act on the findings of evaluation of learning a assessment to develo programmes
		Provide feedbac effectiveness assessme

Midwifery Council (2008) *Standards to Support Learning and* *nt in Practice. NMC Standards for Mentors, Practice Teachers and* *rs*. NMC, London.

INDEX

Note: Page numbers followed by *b* indicate boxes, *f* indicate figures and *t* indicate tables.

A

Absenteeism, 220–221
  evidence, 221
  link lecturer contact, 220
  off-duty review, 220
Accidents, 221
Accreditation of Prior and (Experiential)
      Learning (AP(E)L), 12
Action plans
  failing students, 138–140, 139*t*
  final interview, 159
  midpoint interview *see* Midpoint
      interview
  sign-off mentor role, 173
Activist learning styles, 76, 76*b*, 78
Actors, simulated learning, 236
Acts, definition, 61*b*
ADHD (attention deficit hyperactivity
      disorder), 203
Advance agreements, reasonable disability
      adjustments, 196
Agreement for Reasonable Adjustments, 194
Allocation of mentors, 41
  case study, 42
Annual updating, 14
Anticipatory duty, reasonable disability
      adjustments, 191
Appeals, 213*b*
Applies, definition, 61*b*
Applying for mitigation, 213*b*
Arrival time, student preparation, 38–40
Articles, updating, 16
Assessment(s)
  disabled students, 205–206
  final interview, 149
  final interview failure, 161–164
  ongoing achievement record (OAR), 181
  professional conduct, 217
Assessment book *see* Practice assessment
      document (PAD)
Assessment of practice record *see* Practice
      assessment document (PAD)
Attention deficit hyperactivity disorder
      (ADHD), 203
Attitudinal barriers, disability, 188
Audit trails, failing students, 141

B

Becoming a mentor, 10–12, 11*f*
  qualifications, 10–12
Bereavements, 215–216
Blood-borne infections
  reasonable disability adjustments, 200 *see
      also specific infections*
BSc Specialist Practitioner, 11

C

Cancer, disabled students, 188
Capacity, definition, 40
Care refusal (of student), 227–228
  evidence base review, 227
  note review, 227
  role play, 227
  support role, 227
Case studies
  allocation of mentors, 42
  assessment documentation, 53–54
  conflict resolution, 225
  difficulties in placement, 64
  disabled students, 197
  experience (as mentor), 4
  failing students, 132, 134, 136
  feedback, 92, 93, 97, 104, 116, 134, 245
  feedback sandwich, 100
  final interviews, 152, 156, 157, 162
  initial interviews, 71, 72, 73–74
  learning outcomes, 63, 129
  learning styles, 77
  mentor experience, simulated learning, 253
  mentor records, 17
  midpoint interview, 109, 111, 116, 121
  off-duty planning, 84
  patient visits, 219
  practice assessment document use during
      placement, 56
  pregnancy, 222
  second attempts, 210
  significant event debriefing, 155
  simulated learning, 237, 245, 246, 254
  student expectations, 31
  student, experience as, 2

Certificate in Education, 11
Challenges, 209–232
 definition, 61b
 resources, 232 see also specific instances
Checklists
 final interview, 150
 formal feedback, 96b
 simulated learning, 242b
 student preparation, 48b
Chronic fatigue syndrome, reasonable
  disability adjustments, 200–201
City and Guilds 730/7307, 11
Clinical areas, midpoint interview, 110b
Clinical currency and capability, sign-off
  mentors, 168–170, 169b
Clinical practice, simulated learning,
  235
Clinical skills book see Practice assessment
  document (PAD)
Colleagues
 simulated learning, 240
 support for failing students, 140
Communication barriers, disability, 188
Community placements, 229–231
 diary, 230
 home visits, 231
 patient allocation, 230
 patient contact, 230
 study days, 230
 timetables, 230
Competence assessments, 23–28
 disabled students, 205
 self-assessment form, 24b
 sign-off mentor role, 173
Competence expectations, initial interview,
  82–85
Computer-based simulated learning, 235
Confidentiality
 disability disclosure, 199
 ongoing achievement record
   (OAR), 178
 student complaints, 224
Conflicts
 resolution, case study, 225
 second attempts, 209–210
Consistency, work–life balance, 214–215
Constructive feedback, 98–99
Contact numbers, initial interview, 86–87
Contacts, orientation, 71

Contribute, definition, 61b
Current programme knowledge, sign-off
  mentors, 170

D

Data Protection Act, disability disclosure,
  199
Debriefing, simulated learning
  see Simulated learning
Decision making, final assessment, 212–214
Deferred, 213b
Delays, midpoint interview, 112b
Demonstrate, definition, 61b
Describe, definition, 61b
Developmental framework, 273–284
Diabetes mellitus, reasonable disability
  adjustments, 201
Diaries, community placement, 230
Difficult feedback, 103–105
 case study, 104
 link lecturers, 104
 support, 104
Difficulties in placement, case study, 64
Direct discrimination, disability, 189
Disabilities/disabled students, 185–208
 assessments, 205–206
 cancer, 188
 case study, 197
 categories, 187b
 communication barriers, 188
 direct discrimination, 189
 disclosure see Disability disclosure
 diversity training, 192
 equality training, 192
 feedback, 205
 harassment, 190
 HIV infection, 188
 legislation, 188–191
 medical model, 187–188
 meetings, 205
 models of, 186–188
 multiple sclerosis, 188
 NMC requirements, 191–192
 non-disclosure, 197–199
 physical barriers, 188
 policy barriers, 188
 procedural barriers, 188

reasonable adjustments *see below*
related-discrimination, 189
resources, 207
social model, 188
support evaluation, 206–207, 206*b*
support funding, 194
victimization, 190
Disabilities, reasonable adjustments,
    190–191, 195–196, 200–205
advance agreements, 196
agreement to, 194
blood-borne infections, 200
chronic fatigue syndrome, 200–201
diabetes mellitus, 201
epilepsy, 201
hearing impairments, 201–202
hepatitis B, 200
hepatitis C, 200
HIV infection, 200
learning difficulties, 203, 204*b*
mental health problems, 202
none agreed, 197
sickle cell anaemia, 202–203
thalassemia, 202–203
visual impairment, 203–205
Disability disclosure, 193–200
confidentiality, 199
following actions, 194–195
initial interview, 81–82
late in placement, 196
mentor's responsibility, 195–199
student's responsibility, 199–200
Disability Discrimination Act (DDA)
    (1995), 187, 188
disclosure implications, 193
implications of, 192–193
Disability Discrimination Act (DDA)
    (2005), 189
Disability Team Advisors, 194, 200
Discrimination
direct, disability, 189
related, disability, 189
Discussion, simulated learning feedback,
    252–253
Diversity training, disabled students, 192
Documentation
failing students, 141–142
feedback *see* Feedback
final interview *see* Final assessment

midpoint interview, 120–122, 125
ongoing achievement record (OAR), 178
understanding of, initial interview, 86–87
Drop-in groups (surgeries), updating, 16
Due regard, 20–22
case study, 22
definition, 20, 21
specialist knowledge, 21
Duty times
work–life balance, 214
see also Off-duty times
Dyscalculia, 203
Dyslexia, 203
Dyspraxia, 203

E

Education/practice changes, sign-off
    mentors, 170
ENB 997, 10
ENB 998, 10
Ending phase, final interview, 165–166
Ensures, definition, 61*b*
Entry requirements, register, 36–37
Epilepsy, reasonable disability adjustments,
    201
Equality training, disabled students, 192
Establish, definition, 61*b*
Evaluation, 257–272
environment improvement, 270–272
importance, 257
lessons learnt, 269–270
    mentor misunderstanding, 269
    service delivery, 269
    staff shortages, 269
mentor's experience, 263–266
    guided reflection, 266
    reflection, 264–265, 265*b*
    student questionnaire, 266–269, 267*b*
    SWOT analysis, 263, 267*b*
quality of placement, 259–263
    educational audits, 259–263
student's experience, 258–259, 260*t*
timing, 257–258
what of, 258
Evidence
absenteeism, 221
failing student feedback, 136–137

Evidence (*Continued*)
    final interview feedback, 151–152
    practice assessment document
        consolidation, 65–67
    required, triennial review, 19*t*
Evidence base review, care refusal (of
    student), 227
Experience (as mentor), case study, 4
Explanations, professional conduct,
    217
Extension requests, 213*b*

F

Facilitation role, simulated learning
    see Simulated learning
Failing students, 127–148
    challenges, 127
    consequences, 145–146
        effect on mentor, 146
        second attempts, 146
    definition, 127
    documentation, 141–142
    early vs.late failure, 137–138
    feedback, 133–137
        case study, 134
        evidence, 136–137
        objectivity, 137
        popularity, 136
    final assessments, 142–145
        guilt, 143
        ongoing achievement record, 145
        preparation for failure, 143–144
    final interview *see* Final interview
    help for, 138–141
        action plans, 138–140, 139*t*
        colleague support, 140
        university support, 140–141
    honesty, 142
    initial interview faults, 131
    learning outcome failure, 128–129
        case study, 129
    mentor, effects on, 146, 147–148, 147*b*
    NMC proficiencies, 129–130
    non-avoidance, 128
    problem identification, 131–133
        case study, 132
        over-judgement, 133

reasons for, 130–133
    during placement, 131
    warning signs, 131
sign-off mentor role, 173–174
student denial, 135
    case study, 136
    incorrect judgement, 135
Fair feedback, 105–106
Feedback, 89–106
    assessment, 91–94
    clarity of, 97
        case study, 97
    constructive, 98–99
    definition, 89, 91–92
    delivery of, 96–98
    difficult *see* Difficult feedback
    disabled students, 205
    documentation, 101–103
        ongoing achievement record, 105
        practice assessment document, 103
    efficacy, 90
    failing students *see* Failing students
    failure to give, 93–94
        case study, 93
    fair and honest, 105–106
    final assessment, 95–96
    final interview *see* Final interview
    formal *see* Formal feedback
    informal, 94–95
    initial interview, 95–96
    instigation of, 95
    midpoint interview *see* Midpoint
        interview
    performance concerns, 96–97, 98
    preparation for, 91
    previous experience, 89–91, 90*b*
    purpose of, 92
    regularity, 95
    scheduling, initial interview, 85
    second attempts, 211
    self-esteem, 99
    simulated learning *see* Simulated
        learning
    students, importance to, 91–94
        case study, 92
    timing of, 94
Feedback sandwich, 99–101, 105–106
    case study, 100
    final interview, 152*b*

Final assessment
  decision making, 212–214
  documentation, 158, 159–160
  failing students *see* Failing students
  feedback, 95–96
Final interview, 149–166
  assessment finalization, 149
  case study, 152
  checklist, 150
  content, 151–155
  documentation, 158–160
    action plans, 159
    final assessment documentation, 158,
      159–160
    learning plans, 159
    ongoing achievement record, 149, 158,
      160
    practice assessment document, 154
    progress reports, 158, 159
    reflective exercises, 159
  ending phase, 165–166
  failure, 160–165
    assessment failure, 161–164
    case study, 162
    mentor, effects on, 165
  feedback, 149, 151–152
    evidence, 151–152
    from student, 153
    whole placement summary, 151–152
  feedback sandwich, 152*b*
  key features, 150*b*
  length of, 156
    case study, 156
  mentor reflection, 166
  objective decision making, 158
  people involved, 157
    case study, 157
  personal reflection, 151*b*
  reasons for, 149–150
  significant event debriefing, 149, 154–155
    case study, 155
    working relationships, 154
  timing, 155–158
Finances, 216–217
  difficulties, 216
First attempt, with second attempts,
  211–212
Fitness to practice, 213*b*
5-day rule, 213*b*

Formal feedback, 95–96
  checklists, 96*b*
  warning of, 96
Formative assessment, midpoint interview, 108
Former mentor updating, 15

G

General planning, student preparation, 38–44
Gibbs reflection model, 249–250, 250*f*
*Good Health and Good Character Guidance
  for Education Institutions*, 192
Good Record Keeping Principles, practice
  assessment document (PAD), 55
Ground rules, simulated learning, 241
Group activities, mentor portfolio, 18
Group dynamics, simulated learning, 247
Guilt, failing students, 143

H

Harassment, disability, 190
Health and safety issues
  orientation, 70–71
  reasonable disability adjustments, 190
Health professionals, midpoint interview
  feedback, 119
Hearing impairments, reasonable disability
  adjustments, 201–202
Hepatitis B, reasonable disability
  adjustments, 200
Hepatitis C, reasonable disability
  adjustments, 200
HIV infection
  disabled students, 188
  reasonable disability adjustments, 200
Home visits, community placement, 231
Honesty
  failing students, 142
  feedback, 105–106
Honey and Mumford, learning styles, 76*b*

I

Identify, definition, 61*b*
Incidents, 221
Income, 216–217

Incorrect judgement, student failure denial, 135
Individual Support Plan, 194
  disability disclosure, 199, 200
Informal feedback, 94–95
Initial interview, 71–74
  beginning, 74
    issue checklist, 74–75
  best practice, 75b
  case study, 71
  competence expectations, 82–85
  contact numbers, 86–87
  disability disclosure, 81–82
  documentation understanding, 86–87
  faults, failing students, 131
  feedback, 95–96
  feedback scheduling, 85
  learning styles see Learning styles
  off-duty planning, 84–85
    case study, 84
  ongoing achievement record, 79
  personality clashes, 85–86
  planning learning experiences, 80–81, 83b
    additional experiences, 80–81
    difficulties in, 80
    learning style concerns, 80
  planning of, 72
  practice assessment document (PAD), 59
  practice learning outcomes, 79
  scheduling, 72
    case study, 72
  second attempts, 211
  staging, 73
    case study, 73–74
Inpatient placements, 231
  live mentor lists, 231
  off-duty, 231
Issue checklist, initial interview, 74–75

J

Jargon
  practice assessment document (PAD), 60, 61b
  university, 213b

K

Knowledge and Skills Framework for Learning and Development, 18

L

Learning contracts, practice assessment document (PAD) see Practice assessment document (PAD)
Learning difficulties, reasonable disability adjustments, 203, 204b
Learning environment, student preparation, 33–35
Learning opportunities
  identification, practice assessment document (PAD), 60–61
  student preparation, 33–34, 34b
Learning outcomes
  initial interview, 79
  practice assessment document (PAD) see Practice assessment document (PAD)
Learning plans
  documentation, practice assessment document (PAD), 83–84
  final interview, 159
  practice assessment document (PAD), 82
Learning, simulated see Simulated learning
Learning styles, 75–79
  activists, 76, 78
  activity, 76b
  case study, 77
  concerns, planning learning experiences, 80
  determination, 75–77
  developing of, 77–79
  Honey and Mumford, 76b
  pragmatists, 76, 78
  reflectors, 76, 78
  theorists, 76, 78
Legislation, disabled students, 188–191
Lickert scale, evaluation analysis, 268
Link lecturers
  absenteeism contact, 220
  difficult feedback, 104
  student complaints, 226

Live mentors, 13–14
  lists, 231
Local mentor register, 12–14, 13*t*
  as live mentor, 13–14
Long-arm sign-off mentors, 176–177

M

Maintain, definition, 61*b*
Manage, definition, 61*b*
Medical model, disability, 187–188
Meetings
  disabled students, 205
  first, 69
  second attempts, 211
Memory difficulties, 204*b*
Mental health problems, reasonable
        disability adjustments, 202
Mentor(s)
  allocation *see* Allocation of mentors
  becoming *see* Becoming a mentor
  effects on
    failing students, 146, 147–148, 147*b*
    final interview failure, 165
  evaluation experiences *see* Evaluation
  experience as, case study, 4
  reasons for, 4–5
  records
    case study, 17
    maintenance, 35
  reflection, final interview, 166
  role and responsibilities, 23–28
    second attempts, 211
  student disability disclosure,
        195–199
Mentor conferences, 16
Mentor portfolio, 18–20
  contents, 18–20
  group activities, 18
  performance review, 18
Midpoint interview, 107–126
  action planning, 122–124, 124*b*
    SMART, 123, 123*b*
  case study, 109, 111, 121
  clinical area, 110*b*
  delayed, reasons for, 112*b*
  documenting, 120–122, 125
  feedback, 95–96, 107, 115–118

  case study, 116
  other health professionals, 119
  formative assessment, 108
  length of, 112–114
  location, 114
  planning for, 112
  problems, 119
  progress measurement, 107–108, 119
  purpose, 107–108
  reflection, 117
    encouraging, 118
  responsibility for, 114–115
  seeking help, 124–125
  success celebration, 117–118, 125
  timing of, 108–114
  weakness identification, 110–111
Misconceptions, student complaints, 224
Mitigation, 213*b*
  applying for, 213*b*
Mixed task trainer, simulated learning,
        236–237
Motivation, 223
Motor skill problems, 204*b*
Multiple learning outcomes, second
        attempts, 212
Multiple sclerosis, disabled students, 188

N

Non-disclosure, disabled students,
        197–199
Non-learning environment, student
        preparation, 34–35
Note review, care refusal (of student), 227
Number of students, 40
Numerical problems, 204*b*
Nursing and Midwifery Council (NMC),
        7–28
  disability, views on, 185–186, 186*b*
  disabled student requirements,
        191–192
  failing student proficiencies, 129–130
  policy changes, 7
  sign-off mentor accountability, 172–174
  sign-off mentor registration, 170–171,
        171*b*
Nursing and Midwifery Council Register,
        21*b*

O

OAR *see* Ongoing achievement record (OAR)
Objective decision making, final interview, 158
Objective Structured Clinical Examinations (OSCEs), 17–18
Objectivity, failing student feedback, 137
Off-duty times
  absenteeism review, 220
  inpatient placements, 231
  orientation, 71
  planning
    initial interview *see* Initial interview
    student preparation, 42–44
Ongoing achievement record (OAR), 178–181
  areas of development *vs.* concern, 180–181
  assessment decisions, 181
  confidential information, 178
  documentation, 178
  example, 179, 180*b*
  failing students, 145
  feedback, 105
  final interview, 149, 158, 160
  initial interview, 79
  for sign-off, 178
  sign-off mentor, 172
Online placement profiles, 44–45
Orientation, 69–71
  contacts, 71
  health and safety issues, 70–71
  off-duty organization, 71
  placement environment, 69–70
  staff introductions, 70
  work area, 70–71
Other services/teams, 228
  student preparation, 228
  worksheets, 228, 229*b*
Over-judgement, failing students, 133

P

Participate, definition, 61*b*
Past experiences, 3
Patient(s)
  allocation, community placement, 230
  contact, community placement, 230
  information in simulated learning, 243–244, 244*b*
  refusal of care *see* Care refusal (of student)
  stimulators, 237–238
  visits, case study, 219
Performance concerns, feedback, 96–97, 98
Performance review, mentor portfolio, 18
Personality clashes, initial interview, 85–86
Personal preparation
  simulated learning, 247–249
  student preparation, 35–38
Personal reflection, final interview, 151*b*
Physical barriers, disability, 188
Placement(s), 229–231
  difficulties in, case study, 64
  environment orientation, 69–70
  inpatient *see* Inpatient placements *see also specific types*
Placement assessment document *see* Practice assessment document (PAD)
Planning
  initial interview *see* Initial interview
  midpoint interview, 112
Policy barriers, disability, 188
Popularity, failing student feedback, 136
Positive mentoring, 272
Practical clinical skills, simulated learning, 234
Practice area, student preparation, 30–31
Practice assessment document (PAD), 51–68
  access to, 86
  assessment documentation, 53
    case study, 53–54
  consolidation, 63–66
    evidence, 65–67
    SMART, 63
  definition, 51–52
  evidence, 62
    quantifiable, 62
  feedback, 103
  final interview, 154
  jargon, 60, 61*b*
  key features, 52*b*
  layout of, 52–53
  learning contracts, 54–55
    Good Record Keeping Principles, 55
    space available, 54–55
    specific learning needs, 55

learning opportunity identification, 60–61
learning outcomes, 57–59, 62*b*
  case study, 63
  initial interview, 59
  meaning of, 59
  open/broad, 58
  SMART, 59, 59*b*
  specificity, 58
  understanding of, 64*b*, 65*b*, 66*b*
learning plan documentation, 82,
  83–84
sign-off mentor, 172
use during placement, 55–56
  case study, 56
writing in, 56–57
Practice assessment strategies, sign-off
  mentors, 170
Practice learning document *see* Practice
  assessment document (PAD)
Practice learning outcomes, initial
  interview, 79
Pragmatist learning styles, 76, 78
Pregnancy, 221–222
  case study, 222
  risk assessments, 222
Pre-placement visit, 29–30, 41
Pre-registration programme progression,
  sign-off mentors, 171
Present day, 1–6
Previous comments, second attempts, 211
Previous experience, feedback, 89–91, 90*b*
Prior knowledge, simulated learning, 241
Problems
  identification, failing students *see* Failing
    students
  midpoint interview, 119
Procedural barriers, disability, 188
Professional accountability, 35, 37
Professional conduct, 217–219
  assessment, 217
  explanations, 217
  reflection, 219
  role playing, 217, 219
Professional development, 4–5
Progress measurement, midpoint interview,
  107–108, 119
Progress reports, final interview, 158, 159
Psychomotor skills, simulated learning,
  234

Q

Qualifications, for mentor, 10–12
Quantitative evaluation, evaluation analysis,
  268

R

Ratified results, 213*b*
Reading problems, 204*b*
Reasonable adjustments, disabled students
  see Disabilities, reasonable
  adjustments
Reasons (for mentoring), 4–5
Recognises, definition, 61*b*
Recruitment, 5–6
Referred, 213*b*
Reflection
  exercises, 159
  midpoint interview, 117, 118
  professional conduct, 219
  simulated learning debriefing, 249–250
Reflector learning styles, 76, 78
Refusal of care *see* Care refusal (of student)
Register, entry requirements, 36–37
Regularity of feedback, 95
Related-discrimination, disability, 189
Requests for extension, 213*b*
Required evidence, triennial review, 19*t*
Resources
  challenges, 232
  competition, student crossover
    management, 226–227
  preparation, 44–47
Reviews, *Standards to Support Learning and
  Assessment in Practice* (2008), 8
Risk assessments, pregnancy, 222
Role playing
  care refusal (of student), 227
  professional conduct, 217, 219
  simulated learning, 236
Role preparation, sign-off mentors, 176

S

Second attempts, 209–214
  case history, 210
  conflicts, 209–210

Second attempts (*Continued*)
  definition, 210
  failing students, 146
  feedback, 211
  with first attempt, 211–212
  initial interview, 211
  meetings, 211
  mentor's role, 211
  multiple learning outcomes, 212
  previous comments, 211
  SMART, 211
  theory assignments, 209–210
  university referral, 210
Second first attempt, 213*b*
Seeking help, midpoint interview, 124–125
Self-assessment form, 24*b*
Self assessment(s), sign-off mentors,
    182–183, 182*t*
Self-esteem, feedback, 99
Sickle cell anaemia, reasonable disability
    adjustments, 202–203
Sickness, 220–221
  university contact, 220
Significant event debriefing *see* Final
    interview
Sign-off mentors, 22–23, 167–184
  definition, 22–23, 167–168
  designation, 167–168
  requirements, 168–176, 169*b*
    clinical currency and capability,
      168–170, 169*b*
    current programme knowledge, 170
    education/practice changes, 170
    NMC accountability, 172–174
    NMC registration requirements,
      170–171, 171*b*
    practice assessment strategies, 170
    pre-registration programme
      progression, 171
    supervision by sign-off mentor,
      175–176
  role preparation, 176
  self assessment, 182–183, 182*t*
  student meetings, 177–178
  supervision by, 175–176
  support of others, 176–177
  when required, 168*t*
Sign-off, ongoing achievement record
    (OAR), 178

Simulated learning, 233–256
  case study, 237
  clinical educator, case study, 246
  in clinical practice, 235
  computer-based, 235
  debriefing, 233–234, 249–250
    design of, 251–252
    Gibbs reflection model, 249–250,
      250*f*
    reflection, 249–250
    stress reduction, 249
    timing, 249
  definition, 233–234
  facilitation role, 247–249
    group dynamics, 247
    preparation, 247–248
    student-centred learning, 247, 248*f*
  feedback, 233–234, 249–250, 252–253
    discussion, 252–253
    planning for, 250–252
    positive, 252–253
    sheets, 251*b*
    student views, 252
    video recording, 250
  feedback forms, 244–246
    case study, 245
  mentor experience, case study, 253
  opportunities for, 238–239, 239*b*
  "patient" information, 243–244, 244*b*
  personal preparation, 247–249
  practical clinical skills, 234
  preparation, 238–242
    checklists, 242*b*
    colleagues, 240
    ground rules, 241
    prior knowledge, 241
    students, 240–242
    tool use, 241
  provision of, 235
  psychomotor skills, 234
  reasons for, 234
  student attitudes, 253–254
    case study, 254
  subcutaneous injection, 243*b*
  types, 236–238
    actors, 236
    mixed task trainer, 236–237
    patient stimulators, 237–238
    role play, 236

SMART
  learning outcomes, 59, 59*b*
  midpoint interview action planning, 123, 123*b*
  practice assessment document consolidation, 63
  second attempts, 211
Social model of disability, 188
Space available, practice assessment document (PAD), 54–55
Special Education Needs and Disability Act (SENDA)(2001), 188
  disclosure implications, 193
Specialist Community Public Health Nurse, 20
Specialist knowledge, due regard, 21
Specific learning needs, practice assessment document (PAD), 55
Spelling problems, 204*b*
Staff introductions, orientation, 70
Stages, *Standards to Support Learning and Assessment in Practice* (2008), 8–9, 10*t*
Standards to Support Learning and Assessment in Practice (2008), 7, 16, 17
  definition, 8–9
  disabled students, 192
  feedback documentation, 101
  historical aspects, 7
  midpoint interview documenting, 120–121
  ongoing achievement record (OAR), 178
  requirements, 9–10
  reviews, 8
  sign-off mentor, 167
  stages, 8–9, 10*t*
Stress reduction, simulated learning debriefing, 249
Student(s)
  complaints, 224–226
    academic link intervention, 226
    confidentiality, 224
    misconceptions, 224
  crossover management, 226–227
    competition for resource, 226–227
  denial of failure *see* Failing students
  expectations, preparation, 29–30

  experience as, 1–3
    case study, 2
  failure *see* Failing students
  final interview feedback, 153
  numbers of, 40
  preparation for, 29–50
    before arrival, 29
    arrival time, 38–40
    best-case, 32*b*
    checklist, 48*b*
    general planning, 38–44
    importance, 47–48
    learning environment, 33–35
    learning opportunities, 33–34, 34*b*
    non-learning environment, 34–35
    number of students, 40
    off-duty planning, 42–44
    other services/teams, 228
    personal preparation, 35–38
    practice area, 30–31
    pre-placement visit, 29–30, 41
    problems, 31–33
    resource preparation, 44–47
    student expectations, 29–30, 31
    worst-case, 32
  responsibility, disability disclosure, 199–200
  training programme, understanding of, 36
  views, simulated learning feedback, 252
Student-centred learning, simulated learning, 247
Student-centred simulated learning, 248*f*
Student information packs/folders, 45–46
  updating of, 47
Student meetings, sign-off mentors, 177–178
Student noticeboards, 46–47
Study days, community placement, 230
Subcutaneous injection, simulated learning, 243*b*
Success (in mentoring), 6
Success celebration, midpoint interview, 117–118, 125
Support, 37–38
  definition, 61*b*
  evaluation, disabled students, 206–207, 206*b*
  funding, disabled students, 194
Support role, care refusal (of student), 227

T

Thalassemia, reasonable disability adjustments, 202–203
Theorist learning styles, 76, 78
Theory assignments, second attempts, 209–210
Timetables, community placement, 230
Timing
    final interview, 155–158
    midpoint interview, 108–114
    simulated learning debriefing, 249
Tool use, simulated learning, 241
Triennial review, 18–20
    required evidence, 19t
    timing of, 20
12-week rule, 213b

U

University
    failing student support, 140–141
    jargon, 213b
    second attempt referral, 210
    sickness contact, 220
University and Colleges Admissions Service (UCAS), disabilities, 187
Updating, 14–18
    annual, 14
    articles, 16
    drop-in groups (surgeries), 16
    former mentor updating, 15
    mentor conference, 16

Objective Structured Clinical Examinations (OSCEs), 17–18
workbook/on-line update, 16

V

Victimization, disability, 190
Video recording, simulated learning feedback, 250
Visual impairment, reasonable disability adjustments, 203–205

W

Warning signs, failing students, 131
Weakness identification, midpoint interview, 110–111
Whole placement summary, final interview feedback, 151–152
Work area, orientation, 70–71
Workbook/on-line update, 16
Working relationships, final interview, 154
Work–life balance, 214–217
    consistency, 214–215
    duty times, 214
        case study, 215
Worksheets, other services/teams, 228, 229b
Writing
    practice assessment document (PAD), 56–57
    problems, 204b